Raising a Calf for Beef

Raising a Calf for Beef

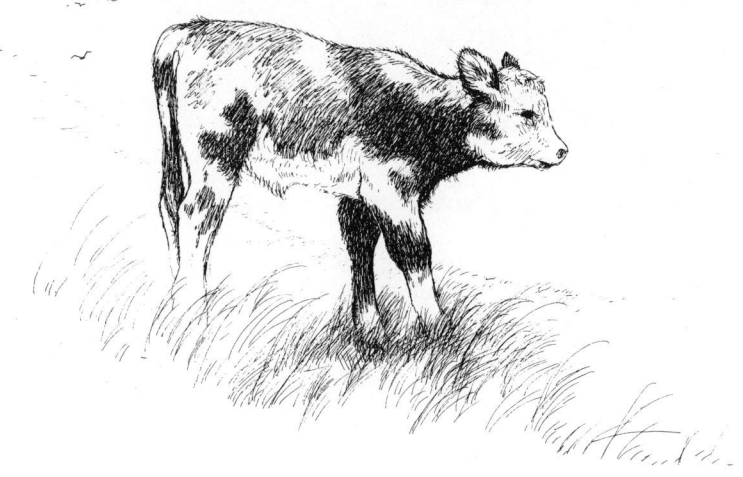

Phyllis Hobson

Garden Way Publishing
Charlotte Vermont 05445

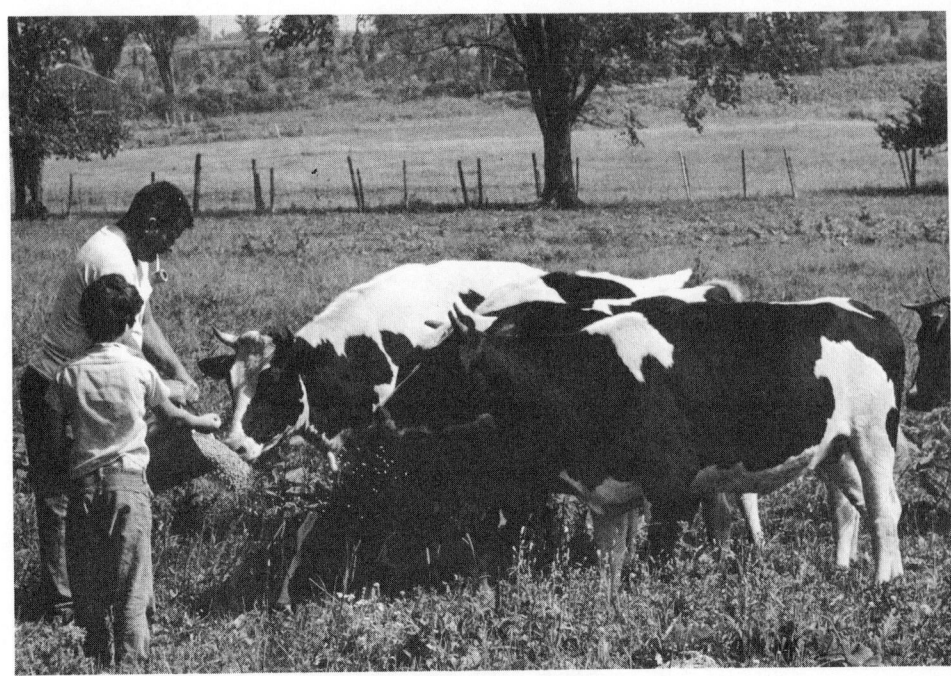

Illustrations By Paula Savastano and Cathy Baker

Photos in Processing Section provided by
The U.S. Dept. of Agriculture

Designed by Bruce L. Williamson

Printed in the United States by Capital City Press
Eighth Printing, April 1981

Hobson, Phyllis.
   Raising a calf for beef.

   Includes index.
     1. Calves. 2. Beef cattle. I. Title.
SF205.H6   636.2'1'3   76-20637
ISBN 0-88266-095-0

Contents

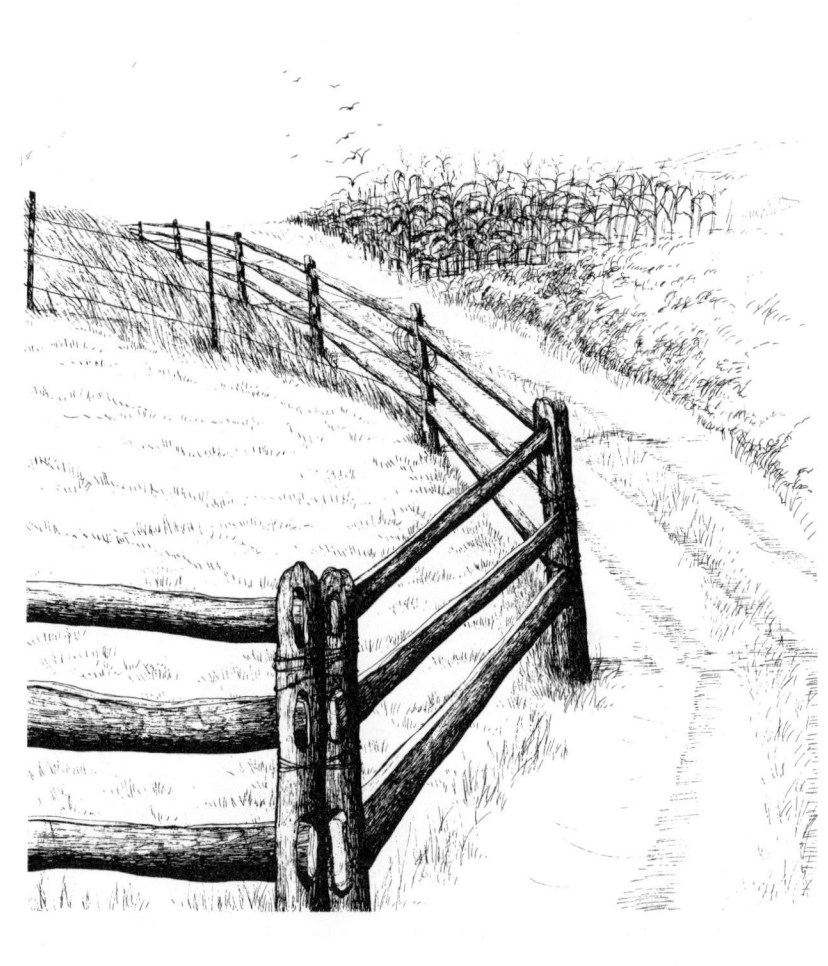

Introduction

Raising a beef calf is an adventure more and more families are embarking upon as they move from the city to a "piece of land" in the country. Initially their reasons may be financial. With the price of food going ever higher, it makes good sense to plant a garden, to can fruit from the apple tree and to raise a calf for beef. But as the project progresses there are other rewards. There is the satisfaction of being self-reliant, of cutting loose from the supermarket syndrome and taking care of one's own by working with nature instead of against it.

And even though there is work involved, raising a baby calf is more of an adventure than a chore. Anyone who has cared for a young animal with attention and kindness, who has watched it grow to healthy maturity because of good care, knows the project brings more satisfaction than just owning a freezer full of meat, more reward than saving money.

But the calf does fill the freezer and it does save money. If you raise your own grain and put up your own hay, you can raise a baby calf for a fraction of the supermarket price of beef. Even if you must buy all your grain and hay, you can raise your family's beef for about half the cost of meat market beef — and you'll be raising better beef. You haven't tasted really good beef until you eat the kind that's been tenderly raised and grain-fed since birth.

So there are at least three good reasons for raising a baby calf: personal satisfaction, financial reward and better eating. That's not even counting the bonus of plenty of garden fertilizer in the form of used bedding and manure.

You may have other reasons. You may have pasture going to waste, an allergy to the chemical preservatives often used with supermarket beef, or you may want to know your meat was grown without hormones or fertilizers or inhuman treatment. Whatever your reason, raising a calf is a good project for the family with a little land, a little time and a little patience to spare.

But it does have disadvantages. It isn't a project you should rush into without considering several points before you buy a calf to raise.

The first is space. Do you have shelter for those winter nights when a baby calf would suffer from the cold, the wind or the rain? An older animal can survive outside in bad weather, although he will suffer if the weather is severe, but a young animal should be kept inside until he is adjusted to his new surroundings and is eating grain well. He also must have shelter from the elements his first winter.

Do you have pasture? A goat, a flock of chickens, even a pig can be raised in a barnyard without pasture to graze, but it is cruel to pen up a calf for a year or two without grass. It is also very expensive, since the calf needs a great deal of green hay to supply the Vitamin A nature intended him to get from a field of green grass.

Do you have the money to invest? Raising a calf should save you money, but it's a long-term investment. It is possible to raise an 800- to 1000-pound calf in one year, but heavy beef takes two or more years. Meanwhile, there not only is no return on your original investment in the calf, but you'll be paying interest in the form of hay and grain every day.

And finally, do you have the time and the patience to teach a small, stubborn animal to drink from a bucket and eat grain from a feeder? Do you want to spend weekend time cleaning his stall? Do you want to go to the barn to feed the calf every day, twice a day, through rain and snow, even when it's below zero or above 90 degrees?

If you do, read on. You're about to embark on one of the

most basic of man's adventures which dates back to early civilization. You're about to become a cattleman.

You'll Need:

Snug, dry housing
Tight fences — Hay
Pasture — Barn bedding
Grain pan — Nursing bucket or bottle
Water bucket — Milk
Hay rack or substitute — Grain
Grooming brush — Lots of patience
Halter — A little time
Mineral box — The healthiest calf you can find

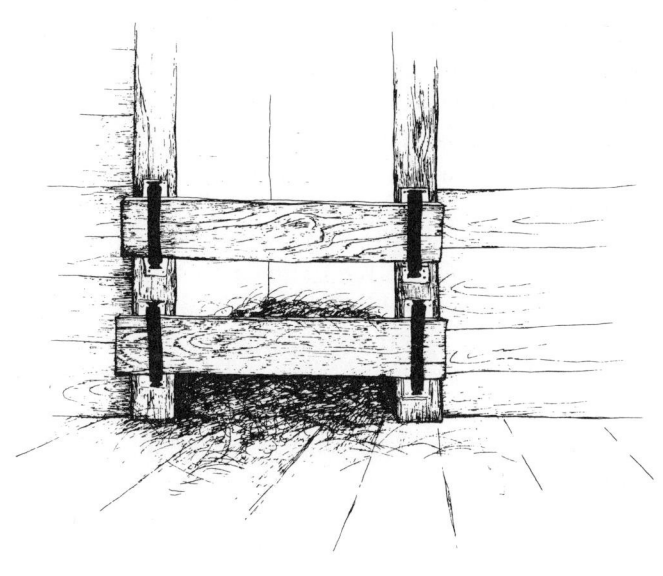

Housing
and Pasture

A baby calf needs shelter. In mild climates it may be needed only for the first few months, and a small, three-sided shed with a pen may suffice during that time. Except in severe climates, older calves may be allowed to stay outside, although they appreciate a dry bed out of the wind and will gain weight better if it is provided.

It need not be a fancy barn. It needn't even be a barn, although a dry, quiet barn corner is an ideal place to raise a baby calf. A shed will do or a barn porch or a lean-to added to the back of a garage. We once housed a baby calf at night in the shell of an old, clean outhouse for a few weeks while his shed was being built, and he liked it just fine. But be sure his housing is dry and snug and free of drafts. A young animal can stand the cold if he is kept dry and out of drafts.

A hand-raised calf should be kept penned up inside for the first few weeks so you can feed him easily at regular intervals and keep a close check on his progress. The pen or stall should be conveniently near, so that you will not hesitate to look in on him several times a day the first few days. Keep him in a building not far from the house and convenient to the water, hay and grain supplies, and a place reasonably easy to keep clean and dry.

Once you have chosen the spot where your baby calf is going to spend his first few weeks, check it for cracks or leaks, for holes and places where the siding has loosened. Patch them with pieces of wood or plug them with caulking. If there are

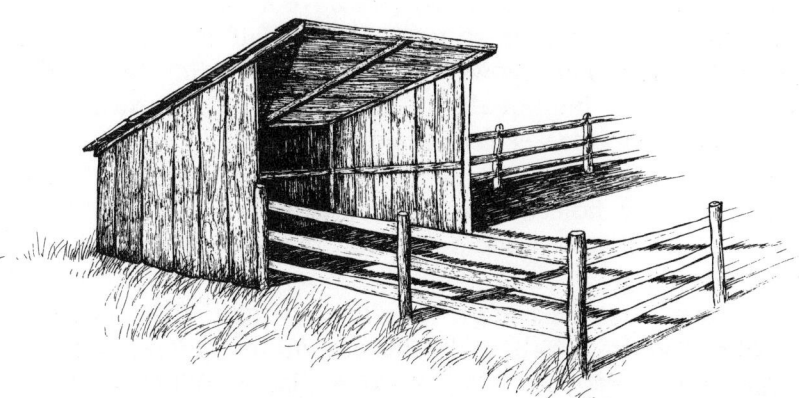

windows, repair them if necessary. In larger quarters you may want to create a snug corner by nailing up stall sides, portable gates or plywood siding.

Check, too, for sharp objects, large and small. Look for pieces of broken glass and bits of cut wire which a calf might swallow. Spikes, jutting pieces of wood or any pointed, splintery places where a small frightened animal could hurt himself should be removed or rounded off.

Now look around at the accomodations. Is there a hay rack low enough for a small calf to reach? Is there a place to hang a water bucket and a feeder? If not, you can construct a low hay rack with scraps of wood. It needn't be fancy. It is even possible to use a metal tub for hay if necessary.

If you're buying a water bucket, get one that hooks on the side of the stall, then hang the bucket and feeder pan at calf height to avoid contamination with manure. If they must be placed on the floor, be prepared to clean them often, for the calf is sure to soil them at least once a day.

Now see that the sleeping quarters are as clean and dry as you can make them. Remove all the old bedding and scrub down the walls, using an old broom or brush and a hot solution of lye water or disinfectant. Let the area dry two or three days, then spread lime over the entire floor. Now lay down about one foot of clean bedding.

How about the pasture? Do you have a minimum of two acres? Is it cross-fenced so you can use half of it at a time while the other half grows? Does it need seeding to insure some clover for high-quality feed? Does it need mowing to prevent undesirable weeds from going to seed?

Are the fences tight? A small calf can get through a surprisingly small hole or over a surprisingly high fence if it wants to. It's better to find a hole now than after your calf has gone through it.

To store your feed grains you'll need tight, dry, rodent-proof containers. Nothing fits this description quite as well as metal, but for economy you could use plastic containers. For small amounts of grain (100 to 200 pounds) a large, clean garbage can with a tight-fitting lid is ideal. For larger amounts you can construct wooden bins lined with thin sheet aluminum or galvanized steel. Excellent, long-lasting bins can be made from discarded galvanized watering tanks by putting wooden lids on them.

You'll also need a water bucket or two, a feed pan, and a nursing pail or calf nursing bottle if you intend to raise an unweaned calf.

You might like to have a curry comb or a brush for grooming, a pick or pocketknife for keeping hooves comfortable, and a calf halter for gentling the calf and for transferring him from one pen to another.

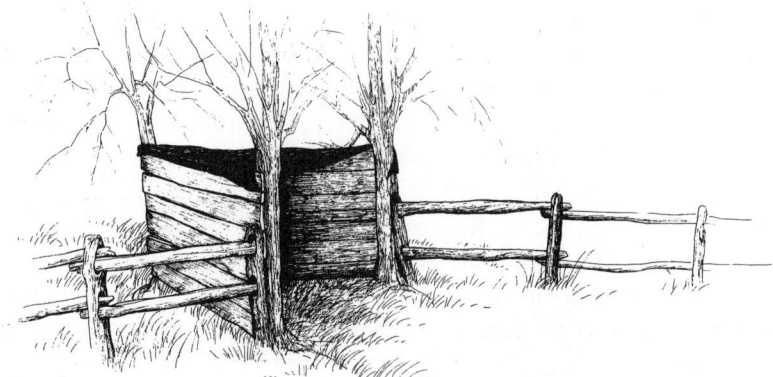

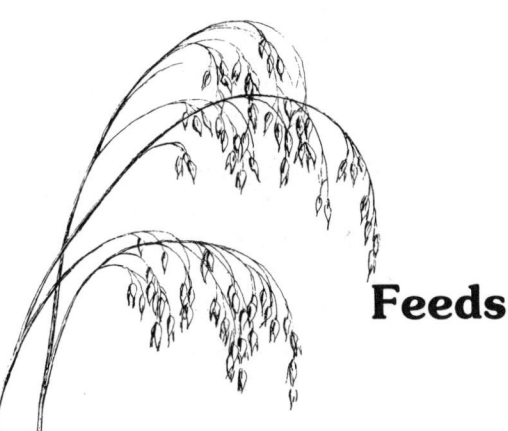

Feeds

Now it's time to stock the larder for your calf. The first year you'll need about 75 bales of hay, more if your pasture is poor and must be supplemented with hay during the summer months.

If you have the land you should plan to grow your own hay, even if you must hire someone with the machinery to cut and bale it for you. Enough hay for one calf may be grown on one acre, especially if you seed it in the spring, and for one-third the price of a good supply of high-quality hay.

If you must buy your hay, arrange to get it in early summer, right from the pasture immediately after it has been cut and baled. It will cost about half as much as winter hay which has been lifted and hauled and stored until the supply decreases and the demand increases. Select mixed clover hay and be sure it is fresh and green. Hay that was rained on after it was cut, or hay that has been stored for a year or more has lost many of its nutrients as well as its green color.

Whether you grow or buy it, you'll have to store your winter's supply of hay in a dry, cool place with good air circulation and out of direct sunlight. Barns usually have several convenient spots that fit this description. If you haven't enough storage area perhaps a neighboring farmer will rent you space in his.

Then you'll need grain. Nothing is as good for a calf as your own grain, grown on your own, enriched soil. You easily can grow enough grain for one calf on an acre or so of land, and harvesting by hand or with simple equipment is not difficult in such small amounts. Lacking that, you can buy your grain directly from a neighboring farmer who grows it, or from a nearby feed store or grain elevator. It's a good idea, if you have the storage space, to have a reserve supply for the crisis of an empty feed bin on a Sunday morning.

You may want to buy mixed calf starter at your local feed store. This starter mix is balanced to include all the grains, protein, vitamins and minerals the calf needs for optimum growth. It eliminates the need for grinding and mixing and adding supplements yourself. But it also includes a great many chemicals and antibiotics in your calf's diet, which may be one of the reasons for raising your own calf in the first place. It also makes it impossible for you to give your calf the nutritional benefits and the appetite-encouraging flavor of fresh-ground grains.

So if you'd like to take the trouble to grind and mix your own, or — even better — if you plan to use your own home-grown grains, here are some approved calf starter formulas. Choose the formula that makes the best use of the grains you can grow or the grains available at lowest cost in your area.

CALF STARTER #1

30 pounds whole, shelled corn
10 pounds rolled or ground oats
10 pounds crushed wheat
10 pounds ground soybeans
 5 pounds bone meal
 1 cup salt
 4 ounces cod liver oil
    or Vitamin A-D and E powder

Shelled corn and rolled oats are available at most grain elevators or feed stores. If crushed (or rolled) wheat is not available in your area, you may substitute wheat bran or buy whole wheat berries and crush them in a hand grist mill, a grain grinder or even a kitchen blender. Ground soybeans may be available at your feed store. If not, you can buy whole soybeans (or raise your own) and run them through a coarse-bladed grist mill or food grinder. Bone meal is available in feed stores or garden supply shops. Iodized table salt may be purchased at grocery stores, cod liver oil at drug stores (in four- and eight-ounce bottles) and Vitamin A-D and E powder at farm supply stores.

CALF STARTER #2

- 25 pounds whole corn
- 30 pounds rolled (or ground) oats
- 8 pounds liquid molasses
  or 11 pounds dry molasses
- 15 pounds wheat bran
- 8 pounds ground soybeans
- 10 pounds non-fat dry milk powder
- 1 cup salt
- 4 ounces cod liver oil
  or Vitamin A-D and E powder

CALF STARTER #3

- 30 pounds whole corn
- 30 pounds whole barley
- 8 pounds liquid
  or 11 pounds dry molasses
- 30 pounds crushed wheat
- 10 pounds non-fat dry milk powder
- 1 cup salt
- 4 ounces cod liver oil
  or Vitamin A-D and E powder

For each formula, mix the grains thoroughly in a clean, shallow bin or a shallow wooden box which you can make especially for this purpose. When well mixed, pour in all eight pounds liquid molasses or two pounds dry molasses mixed with water. Stir until molasses is absorbed. Spread out as thin as possible and let set a few hours, then mix again and store in clean, covered containers. The amount in these formulas will store in a large-size garbage can.

Any of these mixtures is suitable for a calf from a few days to 12 weeks of age. The calf also should have free access to green hay and be receiving whole milk, reconstituted dry skim milk or milk replacer.

All in all you'll need about 3000 pounds of grain to raise a calf to between 800 and 1000 pounds. The first year the calf will require a ton of grain in addition to milk, hay and pasture. The last half year he will need another 1000 pounds. Using the growing table on page 47 as a base, you'll need:

750 pounds (15 bushels) corn	300 pounds (5 bushels) soybeans
750 pounds (22 bushels) oats	450 pounds non-fat dry milk solids
750 pounds (15 bushels) wheat or barley	

After the calf is two or three months old, substitutions may be made for more economical feeds. Although the ratio of corn should be kept approximately the same because of its Vitamin A content and general economy, the other grains — oats, wheat bran, crushed wheat and barley — may be used according to the availability and price of the grains. Dried beet pulp may be substituted for up to one-fourth of the grain. Cane molasses and blackstrap molasses may be used interchangeably at any age. Wheat bran, linseed meal or cottonseed meal may be used to replace all or part of the ground soybeans.

Although the preparation and storage of silage is beyond the scope of most one-calf farmers, if silage is available at low cost it is excellent feed for calves. After the calf is four months old he may be fed six to eight pounds of silage a day with about four pounds of alfalfa hay (in this case preferred over clover) or one to two pounds of grain mixture. The calf should not be fed silage alone without a protein supplement.

It is possible for a calf to live a long and healthy life eating nothing but hay and pasture grass. But it will be four or five years before such a calf reaches his full growth and he will be lean and tough-muscled. This muscling makes for good health but not for good beef. For the beef calf to be young and tender at butchering time, he should be raised to full size as quickly as possible. Although many of the Western calves and almost all of the breeding stock are raised without grain, a calf being raised for beef should be grain-fed from the time he is a week or two old.

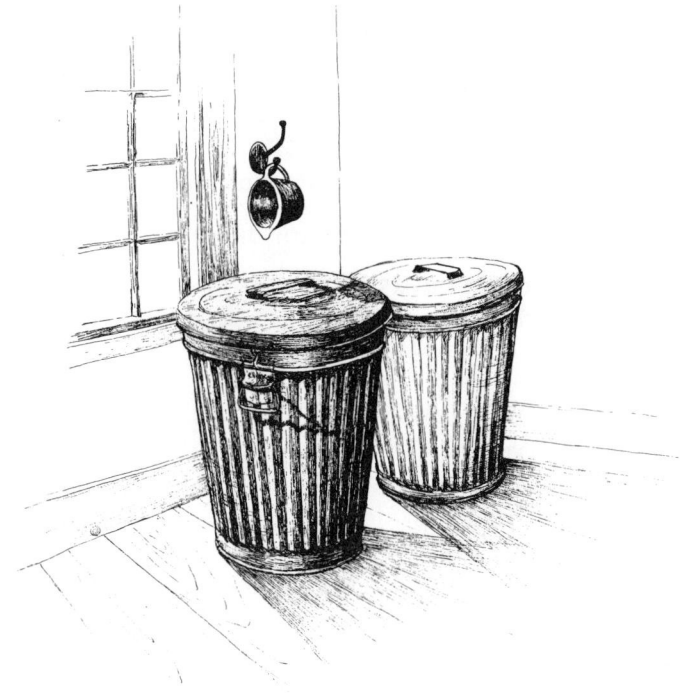

The Milk

A calf less than eight or ten weeks old should have liquid milk fed by means of a nursing bucket or bottle. By far the best milk is that taken directly from the calf's mother. The second best is whole raw milk from another cow. Lacking either of these, you can substitute any one of the following, listed in order of their preference:

Fresh, raw goat's milk, diluted
half-and-half with water

Reconstituted dried whole milk

Reconstituted canned whole milk

Reconstituted dried non-fat milk

Reconstituted dried buttermilk,
diluted by one-fourth with water.

Commercial milk replacers can be used if nothing else is available at a reasonable price. Even then, if possible, start the calf on one of the others and add the replacer to this when the calf is two or three weeks old. When reconstituting, follow package directions exactly.

The following is a good homemade mineral mixture which should be kept available to the calf at all times, either in its stall, or later in the pasture.

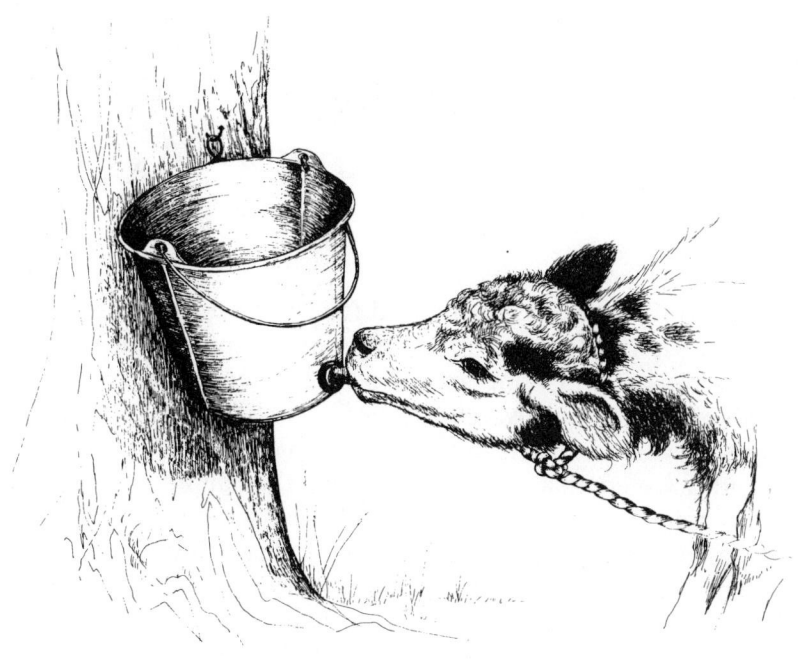

MINERAL MIXTURE

    5 pounds bone meal
    5 pounds ground limestone
  10 pounds salt

Mix well and keep in a small container which is accessible to the calf but protected from rain.

Raising Your Own Feed

If you would like to raise the feed for your calf, you can do so easily with a little time, a minimum of equipment and about two acres of land. One acre should be sown in clover hay. With good weather two cuttings of clover should yield about two tons of good quality hay. Although one person can easily broadcast-seed an acre of clover in less than an hour, it is best to get help at harvest time. If possible hire someone with mowing and baling equipment to cut and bale the hay. Otherwise you can cut the hay with a sickle bar mower, turn it by hand as it dries and store it in the barn without baling.

Since good hay is the most important feed your calf will have, use care in preparing the field for sowing, in choosing the seed and in curing the finished hay. During the winter months, when there is no grass, your calf will have to depend upon the hay you provide for his supply of Vitamin C, so be sure the finished product is bright green and sweet smelling.

Although alfalfa hay has a higher protein content than clover hay, it can bring on stomach upsets when fed as the only source of roughage. Since clover is a high source of protein and easier to digest, a mixed clover hay (i.e. clover mixed with some wild grasses in the field) is best and well liked by calves. It also is easy to grow, easy to cure and safer for the inexperienced. Wild grasses alone may be cured for hay, but the yield is far less, they have far less nutritional value and are not well tolerated by the calves.

A well-fertilized clover field may be cut first in June, just as the clover is in full bloom. With good weather, it may be cut again about six weeks later and in some climates it is possible to obtain a third cutting in the fall.

The second of your two acres should be used to grow the grain your calf will require. Since he will need about 2000 pounds of grain per year you should sow about one-third of an acre each in corn, oats and wheat or barley. In addition, you will need a small plot — about one-eighth of an acre — in soybeans.

The yield from these plantings of grain will feed one calf for one year. If you are feeding several calves, or a combination of other livestock which would require two or three acres of grain, you might be able to hire a neighbor with a combine to harvest your grain crop, but as small a crop as one acre probably would mean you harvest it by hand. In this case, you might be relieved to learn that calves do not require the oats or the wheat to be separated from the chaff. Rough threshing is all that's necessary. The calf won't mind, either, if a little stalk or leaf is included.

In addition to these two acres you will need about two more per calf for pasture, but this land need not be flat cropland. In fact rolling woodland which is unsuitable for crops (maybe with a stream), is ideal for pasture.

By raising the grains and hay your calf will require you will only need to buy the minerals, vitamins and milk. If the calf is on good pasture, the vitamins and powdered milk may be discontinued when he is six months old.

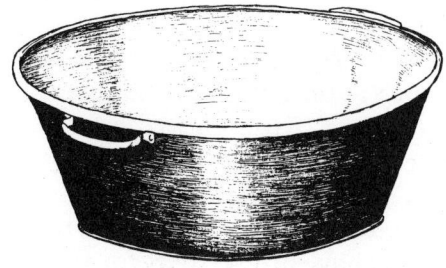

Choosing a Calf

Now you're ready: The calf's quarters are clean and snug and free of drafts. The floor is covered with lime and fresh, dry bedding, and in one corner is a hay rack at just the right height. The winter's supply of hay is stacked in a cool, dark place and you have enough grain for the first few weeks stored in dry, rodent-proof containers.

Now it's time to buy a calf.

What kind you buy will depend on your personal preference, the area in which you live and the amount of money you want to invest. As the old farmers put it, a beef-type calf is more "thrifty" than a dairy-type calf, meaning it will produce more meat for each pound of feed. But the cost of a beef-type calf is considerably higher — enough higher that it might take a lot of corn to offset the difference in price.

If you live in the dairy country of the Midwest, it may be possible to purchase a dairy-type bull calf, unwanted by the dairy farmer, for less than half the price of a beef calf. Castrated while young and raised on grain and grass, these calves — especially the larger breeds — can provide a lot of good beef at low cost.

There is a great variety of sizes among the dairy breeds. Some of these, such as the Jersey, are considered too small and lean to fatten for beef. Holsteins, the largest of the dairy breeds, often are raised for beef because they fatten well, are of large size and have pleasant dispositions. They also gain well on a fairly inexpensive grain mixture. However, because of their height, they have little respect for fences.

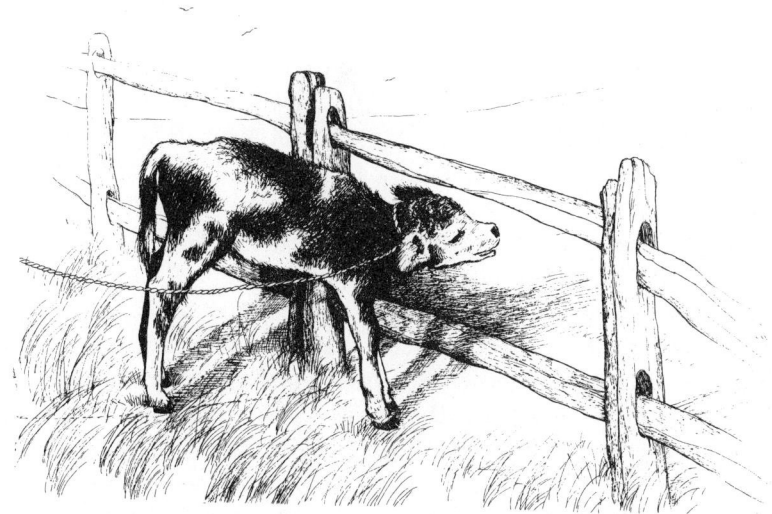

Dairy-beef cross calves are a good choice, because they often retain the fattening characteristics of the beef breed. Some dairymen breed their first-freshening heifers to beef bulls for easier calving. Crossbreed calves are cheaper than beef-type calves, but more expensive than dairy-type bull calves.

If you live in beef-raising country it may be cheaper to buy a beef calf. You may choose from the short, stocky small-boned Angus, the broad-hipped Hereford or the fleshy Charolais. Look around as you drive through the countryside where you live. Ask around at the feed store, the grain elevator. Find out which breed is more popular in your area. That breed not only may be more economical to buy, it also may be better adapted to the climate and therefore easier to raise.

Don't decide on a breed because you like the color or its big, brown eyes. Look around, ask around. Then decide which would be best for you and your pocketbook.

Now you're going to have to decide on age and quantity. Calves are sold at all ages, from a one-day-old, wobbly-legged baby (that needs regular feedings of milk and a great deal of attention) to the six-month-old, well-started calf that needs only a pasture to feed in, plus fresh grain and water everyday.

In between those two extremes there are more than 180 variations, including the three- to five-day-old calf that has gotten a good start from its mother's colostrum but still needs loving care and four to five milk feedings a day. There also is the eight- to ten-week-old weanling that needs no milk — only grain feedings — but requires a watchful eye for any signs of scouring or illness.

Which age you select depends upon your time, your patience and your choice of prices. The easiest calf to care for, the one which requires the least amount of time and trouble — the six-month old — costs the most. The newborn calf, which requires a great deal of attention the first week or two, is the cheapest. In between are the calves which are younger and more trouble than the six-month old, yet older and less trouble than the newborn.

If it's your first calf, the eight- to ten-week-old weaned calf is your best bet. He is still playful and young enough to adjust quickly to new surroundings. In addition, he is still small enough for you to handle easily while you get used to being in charge of a stubborn little animal that doesn't always see eye to eye with you on what you have in mind for him.

A weaned calf is less trouble. He needs no milk, no nursing pails, no nursing bottles. You won't have to go to the barn before you go to bed at night to give him his last bottle of the day. All you need to feed him is grain and hay.

This age also is less risky. The calf already has lived eight or ten weeks, so probably there are no serious congenital defects. He is past the critical stage of his life during which he is prone to scouring. If an eight- to ten-week-old calf looks healthy, he probably is.

Of course you're going to pay for those eight or ten weeks in which someone else — hopefully the mother cow — cared for for your calf. A ten-week-old calf may cost you three times the price of a day-old calf, so the chances are good that one of these years you'll want to raise your own calf, at least from the time he's three days old. But make it next time. This first time you should start with a weanling calf.

It's time now, too, to decide on quantity. Do you want one calf or two or more? Assuming you're interested only in enough beef for your family, one calf would provide enough for a year. But if you like heavier beef rather than the yearling "baby beef," it will take from 18 to 24 months of corn and oats and hay to achieve it. Unless you can somehow make a beef carcass last two years in your freezer, until you can raise another calf, you might want to consider raising two calves at a time.

Besides, calves, like all animals, are much happier in pairs. Unless you have other animals of similar size in the barnyard — goats, a milk cow, a horse or a pony — the calf will get lonely left alone.

One solution is to stagger your calves, always having a young calf and an older yearling. When the older calf is two years old, he is butchered and another baby calf is bought to take his place.

The following instructions assume you'll buy a young bull calf, since the price is usually cheaper and, when castrated at an early age, bull calves grow somewhat larger and heavier than heifer calves. But if you have an opportunity to buy a heifer calf at a good price, especially a beef or beef-cross type, don't hesitate if she seems well-grown and healthy. She will make fine beef, too.

Once you've decided on the breed and age and quantity of calves you'll buy, it's time to go shopping. But the first thing you'll discover is that there is no supermarket for calves. It's a sellers' market and you will have to find the right seller. Here are several sources for buying a baby calf, listed in order of preference:

1. from a nearby beef herd
2. from a neighboring farmer who buys yearling cattle and fattens them in a drylot operation

3. from a nearby dairy farmer
4. from a nearby farmer who occasionally buys 10 or 12 calves, then resells them individually at a profit
5. from a nearby stockyard
6. at a cattle auction

Notice the word, "nearby." That means as close to home as possible. A baby calf is just that — a baby. It needs a warm bed, good food and a feeling of security. However tenderly you care for it, to haul a newborn calf 20 miles or more in a bouncing, drafty truck is to endanger its life. If you cannot buy a baby calf close to home, buy an older one.

Unless you have a calf born on your own farm, your best prospect for a good, healthy animal is to buy one from a nearby beef herd. These calves are bred through generations for beef production and born under ideal conditions, since the breeder usually intends to raise them himself. Probably the calf was born in the spring and dropped in a clean, grassy pasture and has nursed its mother since birth without interference from man. You can't do better than that.

Another possibility, not as ideal but less expensive, is to buy a calf from a farmer who fattens beef cattle in a feedlot operation. Occasionally a heifer being fattened for slaughter will unexpectedly drop a calf. Since the heifer cannot be fattened while she is nursing, the calf must be taken from her. Few men in a feeder operation want to take the time and trouble to raise such an orphan calf, so it is sold or destroyed. If you are willing to try raising a day-old calf that probably has not received its mother's colostrum, give your name and telephone number to a nearby feedlot operator and offer to pay him $10 or $20 for any such calf he cares to sell.

Don't pay much more than that, though. It is possible but chancy to raise a feedlot calf. Unless the operator missed the calf for a day or two, it's doubtful it received that first antibody — colostrum — from its mother. This lack makes the calf a poor risk. If the operator did miss seeing the calf for a day or two, then the calf has been exposed to the stress of overcrowding and the manure and mud conditions of an unsanitary feedlot for a couple of days. Say "no" to a feedlot calf unless it is cheap.

A good dairy farmer usually raises his own replacement heifers, so he breeds for the best. He breeds strong bulls to healthy cows and his calves show it. In addition, they have the advantage of their mother's first colostrum, because his business is milk and he knows the advantages of that first feeding. The calves are taken from the cow at birth and kept in a quiet corner of the barn, but the first three days they are fed the colostrum because the farmer has no use for it in his dairy operation. Besides it is far cheaper than to throw the colostrum away and buy expensive milk replacer. If the barn is clean and the farmer is wise, a dairy calf should be a healthy animal. A farmer who is raising cattle of his own is going to be careful about sanitation for disease prevention. All you have to do is look at his breeding stock to be sure.

In addition to the obvious advantages of buying a calf that has not been exposed to transient cattle and their variety of ailments, buying a calf on the farm where it was born also gives you a chance to look at the calf's mother and judge the state of her health. It's possible also for the farmer who bred the calf to guarantee its health, but you're bound to pay more for a guaranteed calf.

You might be able to buy a good calf from a "calf huckster," usually a part-time farmer who buys 10 or 12 calves for a group price, then immediately sells them singly at a profit. There's nothing wrong with such an operation, but it's definitely a "let the buyer beware" market. Seldom is such a calf guaranteed. But if all else fails, and you can't buy a calf directly from the man who bred it, find a huckster with good reputation and a clean barn and look over his calves.

Of all these sources, only the last one is likely to advertise his wares, and then with a small ad in the local newspaper's classified section. Farmers with good reputations and healthy surplus calves seldom have to advertise. All the calves they care to sell are promised before they're born.

To find them, you'll have to ask around — at the grain elevator, the feed store, the country grocery store. And sometimes the most successful way of all is to drive down a country road until you come to a pasture or a barnlot where you see some healthy looking cattle. Then you just knock on the back door of the farmhouse and ask. You'd be surprised how often it works. If the farmer doesn't have any calves he's willing to sell, he may know of someone who does.

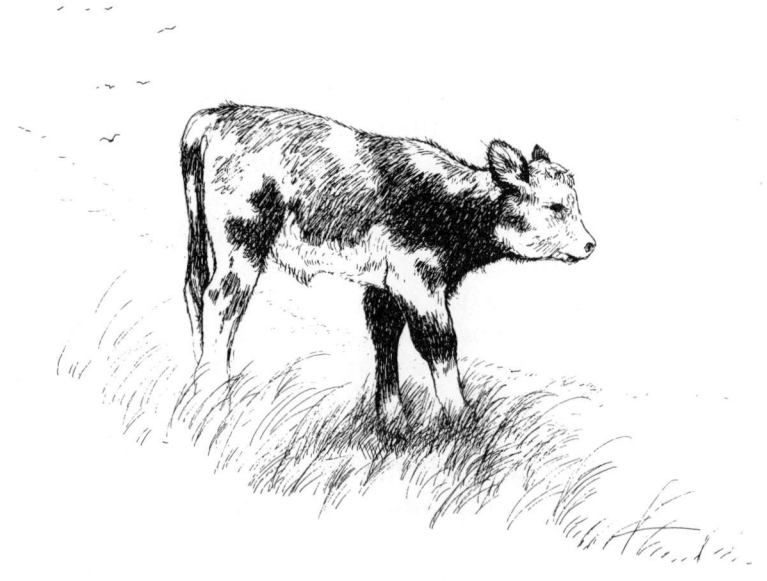

Judging a Calf

How do you judge a healthy calf? First you need to look over a few — healthy and otherwise — to learn the difference. It's a good idea to watch calves in a pasture, to stop by a neighboring farmer's barnlot and ask his permission to look around. And finally, attend a cattle auction or two. You won't become a cattle expert in a few weeks but you can learn a lot.

To judge a healthy calf, look for:

A thick, glossy (or fuzzy) coat. Healthy calves are born with a nice sheen to their coats. If the calf's coat is rough and dull, it may mean the calf or its mother or both are sick or badly nourished, or both. Be wary also of thin or bare patches around the ears or legs. These may indicate parasites. Check for bare patches or a manure-caked rump area, which may mean the calf is scouring.

Loose but not runny bowel movements. Wait for the calf to have a bowel movement. If it's loose enough to fall with a "splat," the calf's digestive system is in good working order. If the stool is hard and lumpy or thin and watery, it would be a mistake to buy the calf. Digestive problems in a young calf can be cleared up, but it's asking for trouble to try it the first time.

Bright, inquisitive eyes and perky, stand-up ears. Dull eyes, a lack of interest in its surroundings and drooping ears are all indications that the calf is sick.

Good posture. A baby calf should hold its head up, its back straight and its tail out a little from its body. A calf that stands with its head hanging, its back hunched up and its tail tucked between its legs is a sick calf.

Personality. At two or three days old a little bull calf will be pugnacious and stubborn, ready to charge any human who tries to force it to do what it doesn't want to do. While little heifers are less aggressive, they will watch human strangers and their activities with interest, and occasionally an especially brave little heifer will approach a stranger. This is assuming the calf is in surroundings in which it feels secure. No frightened animal in an unfamiliar place is going to act as it normally does. But if a calf huddles listlessly in a corner, don't assume it's sleepy or shy. Chances are the calf is ill.

The Stretch. This leaves just one more thing to watch for when you're looking over a baby calf. It's a bit of wisdom handed down through generations of farmers which, though not infallible, is a good sign of health in a young animal: Watch when the animal first stands up after resting or sleeping. According to old-timers, a healthy animal always gives its muscles a good, lengthy stretch before walking away.

The ability to distinguish a healthy calf from one potentially unhealthy takes time to develop — sometimes years.

While your skill still is growing, it's a good idea to ask a knowledgeable friend to go with you when you buy a calf. Lacking such a friend, pay a cattleman or a veterinarian to accompany you when you check over the animals you have tentatively selected. While this may add $10 or more to the purchase price, it could save you $50 or more in the price of curing a sick calf.

Remember the most important day in your adventure of raising a calf, the one that determines more than any other whether the venture will be a success or not, is the day you buy the calf. To make that a good day, never buy a very young calf from a crowded, noisy, hurried place where he has been exposed to heat, cold, wetness, fright and germs from other animals. At best these early stresses can cause a setback that could keep an otherwise healthy calf from ever reaching his potential. At worst, you could be bringing disease, parasites and a lot of work and worry home to your barn. A "bargain" calf is no bargain if he dies or costs twice his purchase price in medical bills.

And don't buy a calf in a hurry. Take your time. Look the calf over carefully. If possible take along a local "expert," maybe even an older 4-H youngster who has raised good calves. If there is any doubt at all that the calf is in top-notch condition, hold off. Look elsewhere. Wait a day. Think it over.

One more thing: Before you buy a calf ask questions. When was the calf born? Does the mother look healthy? Did the calf receive any colostrum? How many days was he on the colostrum? What vaccinations, if any, did the calf — and his mother — receive? What milk or grain is he accustomed to eating now? Don't make a pest of yourself, because the farmer undoubtedly has other things to do, but a few questions and a few observations can tell you a lot about the calf you buy.

If his answers and your observations satisfy you and the "expert" you have asked to assist, it's time to buy your calf. To get him home, put a halter on him and tie him securely in the bed of a pick-up truck or trailer, perhaps even provide a small bed of straw and convince him to lie down until you get him home.

Better yet, why don't you ride back there with him? It will reassure both of you.

Veterinary Help

Unless you already have one, now is the time to select a good veterinarian.

There are two reasons for finding one now: First, make an appointment for him to take care of any routine needs — worming, castrating, dehorning and vaccinations — that you don't feel up to doing yourself; second, to make sure you have a veterinarian who will come in case your calf should become ill. It sometimes is difficult to find one who will come in the middle of the night to treat a patient he has not seen before.

Caring for the Newborn Calf

The amount of time and attention your calf will require depends on his age. A newborn calf will need several visits to the barn a day for the first two weeks. After that, if all is going well, you can gradually cut feedings and barn visits to twice a day.

We'll begin with the care of a newborn calf. If you've taken our advice and bought an older calf, move ahead to the section on your calf's age.

If you're fortunate enough to be on hand when your calf is born, you'll witness one of the most exciting of moments —

the beginning of life. A newborn calf is a limp, wet, helpless, almost lifeless thing until he inhales his first breath, then begins to live and breathe right before your eyes.

If the mother is allowed to keep her calf, she will immediately get to work licking him with her big, rough tongue. This vigorous licking is vital to the calf's well-being for four reasons:

1. To remove the membrane sack in which the calf has spent the past nine months.
2. To dry and warm his skin and make him more comfortable.
3. To stimulate the blood flow which will make the calf warmer and encourage him to get up and walk.
4. To let the baby calf know he is cared for. Even though that tongue may knock him down just as he gets to his feet for the first time, the rubbing is necessary to the well-being of the young animal. It tells him he is loved.

If you take the newborn calf from his mother at the moment of birth, it is important to take her place in this first all-important task. A coarse towel is a good substitute for a rough tongue and the rubbing should be fairly vigorous, but gentle. Rub him all over, thoroughly, to remove the membrane, to dry and warm him, to stimulate his blood flow and to let him know he has someone to care for him.

And while you rub him, talk to him, just as the mother cow does, softly. It doesn't matter what you say. What matters is that he associates a pleasant sound with the person who has now become his caretaker. If you feel foolish talking to a calf — and you shouldn't — then sing or hum or whistle, any reassuring sound he eventually will identify with you. As soon as you have the calf dry and warm, take him to the corner you have prepared for him. There he will spend the next couple of weeks alone.

ONE DAY OLD

As soon as possible dip the still-dangling navel cord in a bottle
of iodine. Swish the bottle around a little, then invert it and
hold it close to the calf's abdomen. See page 50 for further
details. The warmth and moisture of the open navel is an in-
viting place for bacteria to breed, so it's a good idea to elim-
inate these germs as soon as possible.

If the weather is very cold, you should provide some kind of
heat for the first few days, because this is the time when na-
ture intended the young animal to snuggle up to his big, warm
mother. This is another advantage of raising two calves at a
time. They keep each other warm.

A heat lamp is a good, safe source of heat. Hang the lamp
in a snug corner, set low enough to provide enough warmth,
but high enough to keep the area from being too warm. You'll
probably have to turn it off during the warmest part of the
day and you may have to lead the calf to it the first couple of
times, but he'll catch on quickly if he's cold. After two or
three days he won't need the extra heat unless it is unusually
cold.

Does the calf need a little cleaning up? Don't go in for a
complete overhaul, of course, and don't get the calf wet at this
point, but if he was born outside and his coat is caked with
mud or burrs or manure, a small amount of brushing may
make him more comfortable. And, like the rubbing, it is al-
most as reassuring as his mother's licking.

Handle the calf gently as you look him over. Talk to him in
a low, soothing voice. This is a baby you're dealing with. The
sooner he feels safe with you, the better his chances for sur-
vival.

Now the calf has been settled in his new home, his navel has
been treated and he's been cleaned up. He's been rubbed in
that itchy spot behind his ear and he's been talked to. He's
warm and he's been assured that someone cares about him.
It's time to feed him.

If it is at all possible, his first feedings should be colostrum, a thick, yellow "first milk" from a newly-lactating animal. Nature intended colostrum to supply the newborn baby with all the Vitamin A and protein he needs to get him off to a good start, plus enough antibodies built up by the mother to see him safely through the first few critical weeks. He should receive the colostrum as soon as possible after birth.

Since this colostrum is good for nothing but newborn animals, the person from whom you bought the calf may let you milk out the mother for a small fee. One milking from a dairy cow will supply enough colostrum for several feedings if it is refrigerated or frozen as soon as you get it home.

Or perhaps you can buy colostrum from a neighbor who raises dairy cows or goats. A good milk cow or goat will produce far more than is needed for her own offspring. Most dairymen freeze the excess for emergency use.

If you are unable to obtain colostrum, add six egg whites and one teaspoon of cod liver oil to one pint of milk, warm it to body temperature and offer it to the calf in a nursing pail or a special calf nursing bottle. Continue this milk-egg white-cod liver oil formula for two days, reducing the egg white by one egg at each feeding and offering it five times a day at four-hour intervals. The cod liver oil may then be reduced to one teaspoon a day, then discontinued when the calf is eating a satisfactory amount of the grain mixture.

But notice the words "offer it." Remember what I said earlier about patience? Now is the time you'll need it. Even though the calf may be less than an hour old, he knows you're not his mother and he knows that bottle or pail is not his mother's udder. He's not going to walk up and drink the milk you so carefully prepared for him. Chances are he's going to fight you every step of the way. Little bull calves will fight actively, twisting their heads back and forth and backing away from you. Heifer calves will simply clamp their teeth together and refuse to swallow.

To teach a calf to accept the artificial nipple, gently ease him into a corner so he can't back away, then straddle him and force his mouth open, and quickly insert the nipple, squeezing it a bit to give him a taste of the warm milk. You'll have to repeat this several times until he suddenly catches on and begins to suck the nipple as if it were his idea all along.

It may take two or three feedings before he gets the idea, and it will be two or three days before he knows enough to latch onto the nipple by himself. Meanwhile, you'll have to put it back into his mouth each time he loses it.

Be especially careful not to hold the bottle or nursing pail too high. Remember, the cow's udder was placed at the ideal height and it's pretty low. Check each time to see that the nipple is no higher than the calf's back.

In some ways a nursing pail is preferable to a bottle because it can be hung over a rail on the side of a stall once you have selected the correct height. Holding the nipple too high may allow the milk to run into the calf's lungs and lead to pneumonia.

Above all be patient. A stubborn little animal can be aggravating almost beyond endurance, especially when you know — but he doesn't — that his well-being depends upon his doing exactly what he refuses to do. Remember that any tension or loud noise on your part will only increase his anxiety and make him even more frightened and stubborn. Talk to him quietly, handle him gently and, if necessary, introduce the nipple over and over. Eventually he'll get the idea.

The weight of newborn calves will vary from as little as 30 pounds for a small Angus heifer to more than 100 pounds for a large Holstein bull calf. The amount of milk to be given will vary according to the calf's weight. One pint of milk per day for each 10 pounds of calf weight is a good ratio. This means that an average-sized (60-pound) calf should be given about three quarts of milk a day, or two and one-half cups of milk per feeding, five times a day.

Above all don't give the calf too much milk. Overfeeding is far worse than underfeeding for any small animal, and in the case of a baby calf overfeeding almost always is fatal. To be sure you don't overfeed, measure the amount of milk carefully and never give more than the recommended amount at each feeding. A healthy calf always is a little hungry at the end of the milk feeding. Later this hunger will cause him to nibble at — and eventually begin to eat — the mixed grain you will leave him.

Be sure to give him fresh, not-too-cold water every day, beginning with his very first day. He won't drink much at first. You may even have to dip your fingers in it, then let him suck your fingers in order to coax him to taste it. But he will need fresh water, even while he is getting milk, and it is important to have water available when he needs it.

Visit your calf every four hours this first day, each time taking him some warm milk and staying a few moments to observe him and talk to him. Feed him no grain today.

TWO DAYS OLD

On his second day, when you visit his stall, look around for signs of his first bowel movement. If it is a black, tarlike substance all is well. After this first cleanout his stool will be yellow-orange for a week or so, until he is eating grain and hay, but that first black, tarry stool signifies that his digestive tract is in good working condition.

If the first cleanout should be foamy or green or have an unpleasant odor, it is likely that the calf has an infection. You should start at once administering sulfa calf scour boluses, which may be purchased at local feed, drug or farm supplies stores. Administer them by weight according to the directions on the box until the stool is yellow and pasty.

Today, and every day while the calf is confined to the stall, take a minute during your morning chores to clean up his bedding. Take out any wet or soiled straw and replace it with clean, dry bedding. If done daily, this simple routine will take only a few minutes, and it could be more important to your calf's health than all the medicines in your barn medicine chest.   At feeding time, look the calf over for signs of listlessness or discomfort. He should stand up and stretch when you enter the stall, although probably he will still back away when you offer him the nursing pail. He should drink all the milk today, although he may turn away a time or two and then you'll have to coax him into taking the nipple again.

But probably all will be well with your calf this second day and he will be hungry enough to finish his milk at each feeding. Divide his daily ration into five parts and feed him every four hours during the day.

On one of your visits to the barn this day, take a few minutes to brush him. Like the rubbing of the first day, brushing will not only make him more comfortable and stimulate his still-not-quite-up-to-par circulatory system, but also be greatly reassuring to him.

THREE DAYS OLD

On his third day, your calf may meet you at his stall gate with a welcoming "moo." The rattling of his nursing pail, the sight of his nursing bottle, the sound of your voice saying "Good morning" are becoming familiar to him now, and they all serve to stimulate his appetite as he hears you coming. By now he probably can find the nipple by himself without you opening his mouth and inserting it. Probably he is drinking down all his ration and looking for more. Be sure you still are holding the nurser no higher than his back.

Today when he finishes his milk he probably will insist that he needs more. Don't believe him. A baby calf, unlike a baby pig or baby chicken, will kill himself by overeating if allowed to have all he thinks he needs. Today you may divide the daily ration of milk into four parts and feed him morning, noon, at suppertime and again at bedtime. Measure his milk ration in the house and when he finishes it give him some fresh, green hay to nibble on.

Repeat the navel cord treatment with iodine again today.

FOUR DAYS OLD

The fourth day is critical in the life of your new charge. If he was born with more than his share of bacteria or if he inherited an overabundance from his mother, by the fourth day they will have multiplied to the point where they are giving him trouble. Watch your calf carefully on the fourth day for signs of scouring or lack of appetite or just plain listlessness.

If he is scouring but seems otherwise to feel well, cut back on the amount of milk you are giving him. Give him one-third to one-half less. If this doesn't seem to help, add two eggs, yolks and whites, one-fourth teaspoon Kaopectate to one and one-half pints of milk and feed him one-half of this at each feeding for a day or two.

If there is no sign of scouring and he seems to be feeling well, chances are good you have a healthy calf that is off to a good beginning.

Again today divide the milk ration into four feedings.

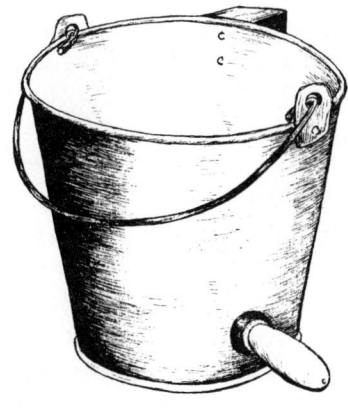

FIVE DAYS OLD

If all is going well two things may happen on the fifth day of your calf's life: He may be introduced to grain and he may start to play.

Teach him to eat grain immediately after his milk feeding. By now probably he has already learned to suck on your fingers. Today before his milk feeding, put a small handful of grain in his feeding pan. Then, as he drinks his milk, take a small handful of mixed grain and tuck a few grains of it into his mouth when he tries to suck your fingers. From now on at each feeding give him a small handful of grain after each milk feeding. By the time he accidentally finds the dish of grain in his stall and begins to nibble on it, it already will have a familiar taste and smell as well as the pleasant association of coming from you.

As for playing, the calf will learn this on his own. Little heifers will flit around shyly, running from one side of the pen to the other. Even at this age little bull calves are more aggressive, sometimes pawing the earth in mock anger, often attacking your knees.

Notice how the calf sleeps in his pen, with his forelegs tucked under his chest like a cat and his head twisted around to rest on his back. Uncomfortable as this position may seem, it is normal for a calf. It is unusual — even dangerous — for a calf to lie on its side and stretch out its legs and neck, because from this position fluid from the stomach can enter the lungs and lead to pneumonia.

Notice, too, how your calf stands and walks. Is its back straight? Does it limp? Unless he has injured himself, a calf that suddenly starts limping probably has a manure ball in his hoof, and it should be attended to before the problem becomes serious. To remove these small lumps of hardened manure or small rocks from a calf's hoof, straddle his leg so the calf is to your back, then bend the leg so you can see the underside of the hoof. With a hoof pick or a dull knife, scrape it clean down to the white, removing any soft, spongy material or foreign bodies. It's a good idea to spray with an iodine solution to help toughen the hoof and discourage hoof rot.

Continue to observe your calf and keep him on the four-feedings-a-day schedule.

SIX DAYS OLD

By the sixth day your calf should be nibbling at the grain in his dish and eating a little hay between milk feedings. If he is eating and feeling well you can divide his milk ration into three parts, feeding him morning, noon and evening and eliminating the final night feeding.

Don't let up on your surveillance, though. Check your calf every time you go to the barn. Look him over. Is he standing straight, or is his back humped and his head down? Is his belly nice and rounded, not flat or concave, not puffed with bloat? Are his stools light colored and of a soft but not watery consistency? Are his ears warm but not too warm? The normal temperature of a healthy calf is 101 degrees. When it goes above this his ears are noticeably hot to the touch.

If you can answer all these questions affirmatively, probably your calf is doing well. Continue to keep his pen clean, control his milk intake and watch him carefully.

But you can begin to relax a little.

SEVEN DAYS OLD

By the time your calf is a week old, he should be able to get along without the heat lamp, even in cold weather, provided his bed is dry and without drafts. Wait until a day when the sun is shining and the temperature is above freezing during the warmest part of the day. Then turn off the heat lamp and provide an extra supply of dry bedding for the night.

Continue with the three feedings a day schedule. After each feeding offer the calf a small handful of grain, rubbing it against his nose and inserting a few grains in his mouth, then leave a cup or two in his feed pan. Keep fresh hay before him at all times.

EIGHT DAYS OLD

By the eighth day your calf may be beginning to ruminate. Since this is all-important to his future health, it is a happy sight to see the small calf lying in his stall, forefeet tucked under his chest, contentedly chewing his cud.

By now your calf probably has learned to stand quietly for his brushing, enjoys an occasional scratch under the neck and around the ears. As you brush him, check for any bare spots, especially around the ears, neck and hind quarters. This could be a symptom of lice or itch mites. Although you cannot see mites, you should lightly dust such bare spots with rotenone.

NINE DAYS OLD

Each morning, as you enter the barn or shed that is your calf's home, use your sense of smell as well as your sight to check on his well-being. Smell can tell you — long before you can tell by looking — when something is wrong. Put your nose in the air and smell. As you enter his stall, again smell. Is there a different odor today? A sour smell, a foul smell?

Sour-smelling feces may mean something is amiss, from simple overfeeding to a serious infection, for fresh calf manure should have a not-unpleasant odor. Foul-smelling breath is a sure sign of serious trouble since the breath of a corn-fed calf usually has a sweet, wholesome odor.

If a bad odor is caused by neither of these, check his hoofs. Hoof rot — caused by the same bacteria which cause calf diphtheria — gives the soft part of the hoof a very foul smell.

Continue giving the calf milk feedings and grain and hay three times a day.

TEN DAYS OLD

At ten days old your calf is ready to go on a two-feedings-a-day schedule. Now you may divide his daily milk ratio into two parts, to be given 12 hours apart.

Each time you go to the barn for a feeding remove any hay and grain left from the previous feeding. (The chickens will be glad to have it.) Put enough fresh, green hay in the hay rack and enough fresh grain mixture in the grain dish to last until the next feeding without having too much to discard next time.

Do all this before you give the calf his milk feeding. Then immediately after he drains his milk pail or bottle, while he is still searching for more milk, insert a little grain mixture into his mouth and lead him to the grain dish. Soon he will go directly from the milk feeding to the grain feeding without your help.

Although weaning time is still another six or eight weeks away, teaching him this little routine now will make weaning infinitely easier. At weaning you will simply eliminate the milk feeding step and the calf will go directly to the grain feeding.

Since the tenth day is another milestone of sorts, look your calf over carefully today. When he finishes the milk feeding stay around a few minutes to bring him fresh water, and clean up his bedding a little. Watch to see if he goes directly to the grain and how much he eats. Is he eating all the hay you put out for him? Does the mineral box show signs that he has been licking it? How does he look? Is he growing? How does he act — is he playful and friendly?

Get in the habit of looking your calf over critically at every feeding. By noting small changes while they are still small you can avoid major problems.

Increase his grain and hay feeding each day as he begins to eat more. He may have two to three cups of grain per feeding now.

ELEVEN DAYS OLD

You should be able to tell by now whether your calf is doing well on the particular milk you chose for him. If it is his mother's milk, nature has taken care of the problem for you. There is no doubt that it agrees with the calf. Probably there is no problem if you are able to feed whole, raw milk directly from another cow.

But if you've had to make a substitution you may begin to notice problems. The most common difficulty is quantity. If a calf appears otherwise healthy yet persists in scouring, the problem undoubtedly is the milk. Either he is getting too much or the milk is too rich.

The first step to correct this is to cut down the amount by one-third. Nine times out of ten the scouring will clear up miraculously with this simple step. If not, dilute the cut-back amount one-third with water, then measure out the usual daily ration. Do not give the calf a larger amount than he has been getting.

If neither of these works, you may have to try a different milk. Our next choice is non-fat dry milk, reconstituted according to package directions, then fed according to the usual ration.

As with any new feed, introduce the new milk gradually, first mixing it half-and-half with the familiar milk for the first feeding or two. This gets the calf used to the change in taste and his stomach used to the new substance.

There are other milks you may try, according to your and the calf's preference, the cost and availability in your area. Raw, skimmed milk where it is available, sometimes may be an inexpensive, easily digestible calf feed. So is powdered or fresh buttermilk, a milk form often more easily tolerated by the calf, although it loosens the stool a little, and he will have to learn to like the taste. Also there are the milk substitutes made especially for calf feeding, although these must be used very carefully according to the package directions.

Lastly, if all else fails, you may have to eliminate digestive problems by eliminating the milk. When a calf consistently has digestive problems on milk you may have to wean him as early as possible. Weaning as young as two or three weeks old sometimes may solve the problem.

If your calf is doing well on milk, continue the two milk feedings a day, increasing the grain and hay feedings as needed.

TWELVE DAYS OLD

You can best judge the state of your calf's well-being by looking at his eyes. A healthy calf's eyes should be clear and bright, the iris dark, the white very white. They should be inquisitive and expressive. Watery eyes may indicate a sensitivity to the dust of hay or grain in his feed pan. It may be a sign of pinkeye or a head cold, or it may indicate a more serious illness.

To eliminate the possibility of dust irritations give the calf only the leaves of fresh, green hay and feed him whole grains with pelleted supplement, or dampen his grain mixture with molasses.

Pinkeye is not only a disease but also a symptom of allergies, caused by flies which irritate the corners of the eye, by contagious bacteria or by a deficiency of Vitamin A.

Whatever the cause, the result is eyes that water, then become red and irritated. There is even the possibility of blindness. At the first sign of watering, the calf's dosage of cod liver oil should be increased by one-half and his eyes should be treated with a boric acid solution, with antibiotic eye drops or an ointment available at any farm supply store.

If you don't have time for a thorough check of your calf

each time you feed him, take a second to check his eyes. After you become accustomed to their bright inquisitiveness, you'll quickly learn to read the message they can give you about his health. Red eyes may indicate a fever or an infection. Dull eyes may say your calf is seriously ill. Sad eyes can tell you — better than any other symptom — that your calf doesn't feel well.

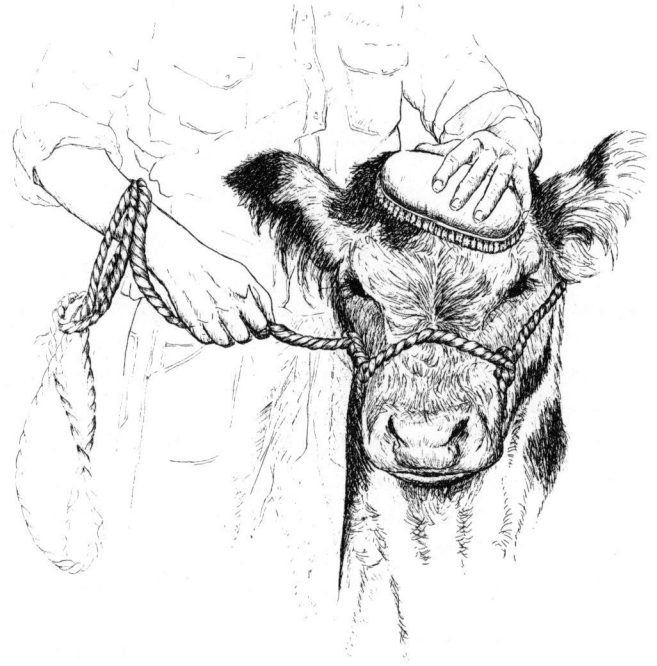

THIRTEEN DAYS OLD

So far we've only discussed the problem of raising a calf in cold weather. It's time to talk about the biggest warm weather problem — flies.

Flies are more than just a nuisance. They carry disease, they winter over in the warm, manurey recesses of your calf's bedding and they can aggravate him enough to stop his gaining properly. Worse, flies can lay their eggs in small openings on the calf's body — in small cuts or in the rectal or vaginal openings — and the fly larva that hatch and feed in those areas can cause discomfort and serious illness.

So it is important to keep the fly population to a minimum. It also is important to do so without using poisonous sprays which would contaminate the calf's feed and bedding and possibly cause respiratory problems.

Some of the simplest, safest fly control measures are the old-fashioned cone-shaped fly traps to which flies are lured by a sweetened bait, the dangling rolls of fly paper and the poisoned sugar-bait which is spread out in high places. All are effective but must be kept out of the reach of the calf and small children.

By far the most effective fly control is a regular program of sanitation. Flies cannot multiply in a barn that has no dirty bedding or manure piles in which to breed.

FOURTEEN DAYS OLD

This is the big day. Your calf is two weeks old, and we hope all is going well. He is eating and growing well. He's acting healthy and has adjusted well to his new home. You've looked forward to this day with both pleasure and dread. It's time to let your calf outside.

This is an important day for your calf, too. Not only will he find it pleasant to escape the confinement of the stall, but he will get his first experience at running and playing in the warm sunshine. And if there is pasture he will begin to learn his life's work — grazing.

It will also mean less work for you. Since his stall will be used only at night from now on, it will require less cleaning. As soon as he begins to eat grass, the calf will need less grain and, eventually, less milk. This day marks the beginning of the end of your role as the calf's constant caretaker.

But you can't help worrying that once you turn him loose, you'll never see your calf again. It's obvious that once you open that door and let him out into the big pasture, you'll have no way of getting him back.

But that's not true. By now the calf is attached to his nursing pail, his warm place in the barn and you — in that order. You and that pail are his mother. He's not going to go off and leave you yet.

So let him out and keep an eye on him for a while, especially if there is other livestock in the pasture. But don't worry about him coming in at night. When he sees you heading for the barn, his nursing pail or bottle in hand, he'll be eager to go back inside to the comfort of his stall and his evening meal.

This will be your schedule for the next six to eight weeks, weather permitting. Each day he will go outside to the pasture and each evening he will return to his pen or stall to have his milk feeding, his grain and hay and to spend the night. In just a few days, he'll get used to the new routine.

Don't be in too big a hurry to let him out in the mornings, though. After he drinks his milk, give him some time to eat his fill of grain and hay. Calves are very slow eaters. Then, an hour or so after breakfast, after the sun has dried the dew or the frost off the grass, let him out.

THE NEXT EIGHT WEEKS

You now have a started calf. He's only two weeks old, he's still several weeks away from weaning and he's far from ready to be on his own. But if all has gone well up to now, your calf is on his way, and both of you have settled down into a routine.

The routine should be a regular schedule which doesn't vary much from day to day. Calves, like all young animals, have a biological timepiece inside them which is more accurate than any clock. They are such creatures of habit that they can become physically upset if their routine gets out of kilter. Just as with humans, they feel more secure if they know what's going to happen next.

For the next six to eight weeks, keep your calf as close as possible to the routine you have set up. Here is one that works well if it fits your own schedule:

7:00 AM: Give him half of his daily milk ration, followed by his regular grain and hay feeding. Give fresh water, then leave him alone.

8:00 AM: Check calf over quickly and, before letting him out for the day, be sure he has eaten some grain and hay. If he hasn't, or if he doesn't seem to be feeling up to par, keep him in his stall where you can make more frequent checks on him. If the weather is wet or windy or very cold, provide him with shelter outside or keep him inside until the warmest part of the day.

12 NOON: Check on the calf. Make sure that fresh water is available and thawed, and that the calf is not being mistreated or kept from the water or shelter by larger animals. If grass is sparse, give him some hay.

6:00 PM: Ready his stall for the calf's return. Top with a handful of fresh bedding if needed. Empty, clean, and refill the water, hay, and grain containers. Then let the calf back in (by now he's probably bawling at the door), and let him have the other half of his daily milk ration. Brush him a little, talk to him a bit, observe the state of his health. Then tell him goodnight and leave him until morning.

Weaning Your Calf

If you have followed our suggestions, your calf is eating two or three cups of grain per feeding, he is eating hay and nibbling grass in the pasture, he is getting no more than the recommended amount of milk in two daily feedings. Now he is a well-adjusted, contented calf, and there should be no problem in weaning him.

The age to wean depends on the calf and your milk supply. If he is big, growthy, aggressive and healthy, if he starts in on his grain the minute it's offered him and eats his hay well, probably you can wean him at eight weeks. But if he is small or has had problems, if he just doesn't seem to care for the grain, or if you have a plentiful milk supply, there is no pressing reason why he should be weaned until he is 10 to 12 weeks old. Beef calves kept with their mothers on pasture often are nursing until they are removed at six to eight months. Let your judgment and the calf's condition be your guide.

Actually, you began the weaning program way back when you divided his daily milk ration from five feedings a day to four a day. Later you introduced other feeds — hay, grains and grass — and little by little you cut down on the number until presently he is getting two milk feedings a day.

Now comes the next-to-the-last step — cutting down to only one milk feeding a day. But there is a change in procedure. This time you won't be giving the same amount of milk per day divided into fewer feedings. This time you will actually be cutting his milk intake in half.

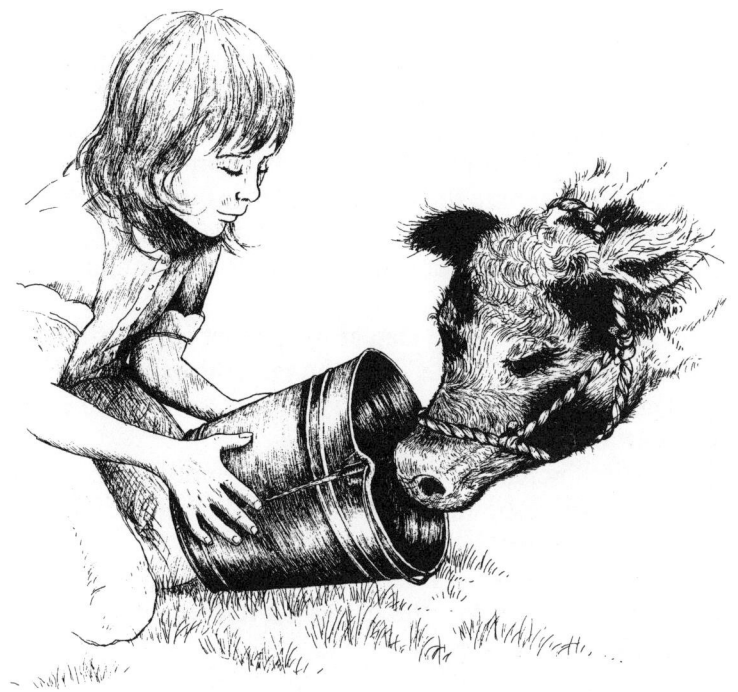

Start with his morning feeding, since he soon will be distracted by going outside to play and graze in the pasture. Just go to the barn at 7:00 as you have been, give him fresh water and hay and grain, talk to him softly for a minute when he bawls his displeasure and then leave him alone to eat his grain. Probably when you go back out at 8:00 to let him out, he will have forgotten about missing the milk feeding. If not, or if he refuses to eat his grain but shows no sign of illness, let him out as usual.

Check on him at noon, being sure he has plenty of fresh water to drink, since he missed the liquid of his milk in the morning. If he is still complaining, hand-feed him a little grain.

At 6:00 PM, return to the usual evening barn routine, giving him his one milk feeding of the day and maybe spending a minute or two longer than usual with him if he seems very unhappy. Probably the milk feeding will pacify him for the night.

After two or three days, he will accept the new routine without complaint. Continue the one-bottle-a-day schedule for two weeks, then eliminate the night milk just as you did the morning feeding, offering instead his usual grain and hay, plenty of fresh water and maybe a little more of your attention for a few days.

If you have taken each step at the proper stage of the calf's development, have made each change gradually and treated him with patience and kindness, you now have a well-started, sturdy little calf.

Gradually increase the grain allowance until the calf is eating two to three pounds (measure in a small coffee can) a day. Divided into two feedings, this would be one to one-and-a-half canfuls at each feeding. When the calf is six months old the grain ration may be increased to four or five pounds per day, according to his size.

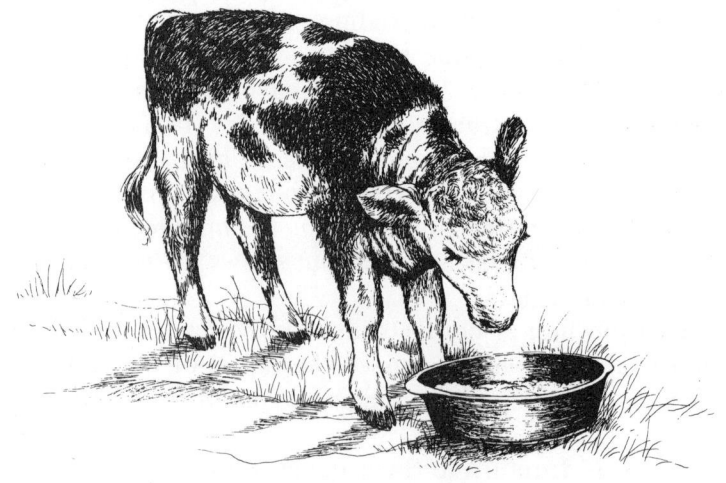

A Growing Ration

After weaning, the calf should be fed a ration especially mixed for growing calves. If you plan to mix your own, here is an approved formula for a weaned calf that is on unlimited pasture or receiving plenty of bright green hay.

30 pounds crushed or coarsely ground corn
30 pounds rolled or ground oats
30 pounds rolled or ground wheat or barley
10 pounds ground soybeans
20 pounds dried skim milk or buttermilk

If pasture is sparse and hay is not of good quality, four ounces of cod liver oil or Vitamin A-D and E powder should be added. Molasses is not needed but may be added for appetite appeal.

Gradually change his grain feeding to the new formula by introducing a small amount into his grain mixture, then increase it each day until he is receiving all of the new mixture and eating it well. Take your time, and make the changeover very gradual. Calves often will go hungry rather than accept a new feed.

Your calf will be going outside every day now, even in very cold weather, provided there is an open shelter available for him in the pasture or barnlot. Be certain there is fresh, thawed water, salt and some form of minerals where he can get to them during the day. The formula for a salt-mineral mixture on page 13 may be used throughout his life. During warm weather, if grass is plentiful, he will not need hay but should be kept on grain.

How Much Time?

Barring any illnesses, from now until butchering time your calf will need less than half an hour a day of your time — 10 minutes in the morning, 10 minutes in the evening and about 20 minutes once a week to clean his stall.

The Barn Medicine Chest

Let's hope that you buy a calf so healthy and take care of him so well that he never has serious problems, and you never have to call a veterinarian. Even so, you should have some of these home remedies in your barn medicine chest:

A bottle of *Kaopectate* or *Pepto Bismol,* for simple scours or digestive upsets.

A can or two of *electolyte,* a liquid product made for children recovering from diarrhea, to replace important minerals lost in scouring.

A box of baking soda, for simple stomach upsets.

A few calf scour boluses, for more serious scouring and digestive complaints. These are available in farm supply stores and are most effective if used immediately.

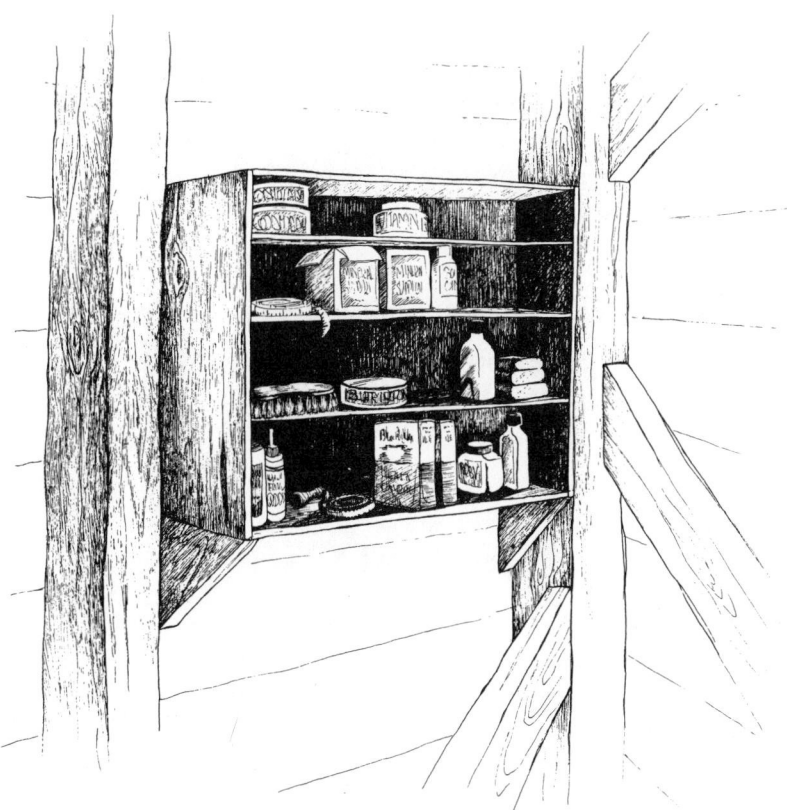

A bottle of diluted iodine spray, for toughening and disinfecting sore hoofs and scratches. You can buy the spray or make it by diluting drugstore iodine (1 part iodine to 10 parts water) and using it in a spray bottle.

A box of epsom salts to be diluted in warm water, for soaking sore hoofs and muscles.

A small bottle of boric acid solution (½ teaspoon boric acid dissolved in one cup warm water), for washing mattered or watery eyes.

A small jar of pine tar salve or commercial udder balm, for fly protection and soothing small sore places.

A quart of fly repellant, made by combining one quart of clean unused motor oil with two ounces liquid camphorated oil. Mix well and rub on the calf's back, belly and head. It is easiest applied while wearing a pair of cotton gloves. Saturate the palm of the gloves with the oil, then rub it on the calf, being careful not to get the oil in his eyes.

A small bottle of aspirin for reducing fever.

A bottle of cold tablets for sniffly noses.

A bottle of camphorated oil for eradicating ear mites or relieving congestion from a cold.

Medical Care

Calves are naturally sturdy little animals, and if you bought a healthy baby, have kept his quarters and his equipment clean, if you have fed him regularly without overfeeding, if you have treated him with kindness — then you probably will never have to treat him for illness. But there are routine treatments you or your veterinarian will need to take care of. They aren't difficult and most of them require no skill or training, but they are necessary.

The first treatment your calf needs is coating the navel cord — inside and out — with iodine. The cord is the fragment of what once was the lifeline between the calf and his mother. Immediately after birth it was severed, leaving a few inches attached to the calf's abdomen, and now it is dragging in the manure of a barn stall every time he lies down. Through it are traveling some pretty bad germs, which will thrive and multiply in that warm, moist place.

In a few days the tube will be sealed off, and the germs

will not be able to enter the calf's body. In a few weeks it will dry up and slough off. But in the meantime you should eliminate as many of those germs as possible.

To do this, lay the calf on his side and drop the cord inside a small bottle of iodine. Then invert the bottle firmly against the calf's abdomen and slosh it around a little. Repeat this treatment in two days.

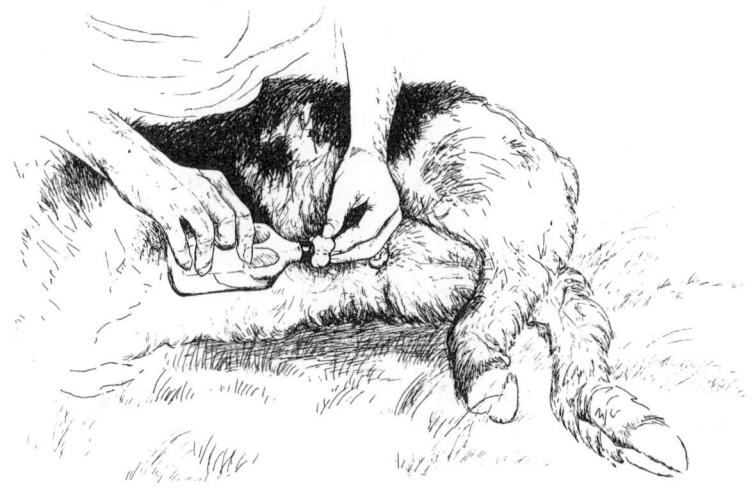

Castration: If you are raising a bull calf for meat, you should castrate him at about two months of age, or as soon as both testicles have descended into the scrotum. The castration can be accomplished in any of several ways, but the only one which should be attempted by the novice is the *elastrator* method.

The elastrator is a metal hand-instrument by which small rubber, donut-shaped rings are stretched to fit around the scrotum; then with both testicles through the rubber ring, pressure is released, allowing the ring to constrict. There is no cutting and no bleeding. The tightness of the rings cuts off the blood supply and the testicles eventually wither and are sloughed off. The calf suffers a slight discomfort the first hour or two, but if the ring is correctly applied there is no pain and he soon forgets about it.

Castration also may be accomplished by surgery or by crimping the blood vessels to the testicles, but these are methods best used by a trained operator or a veterinarian.

Dehorning: Although many calf-raisers never dehorn their animals, others believe it is necessary for the safety of their caretakers and other animals. If you wish to dehorn your calf, there are several methods.

When the calf is only a few days or a few weeks old, just as his horn buttons begin to emerge (the age varies with the breed), he can be disbudded with an electric dehorner or a caustic paste or stick. After the horns have developed, they may be removed by the use of the elastrator rings or surgically cut off.

Any of these treatments may be successful when done by someone with experience, but all are dangerous if done incorrectly. Unless you have experienced help it's best to call upon a good veterinarian to do the dehorning.

Vaccinations: Whether or not your calf should be vaccinated against *black leg, calf diphtheria, leptospirosis* or any other disease prevalent in your area (and at what age it should be done) is a good question to ask your veterinarian when you first contact him. Some calves raised alone are never vaccinated. In other areas it is risky not to.

Worming: Ask your veterinarian about worming, too. While it is possible to buy dozens of de-worming tablets and capsules and powders — and it is a simple matter to administer any of them — without experience or training it is impossible to know which treatment your animal needs, if any. Since all worming medications are poison, calves should never be wormed routinely without evidence that they have worms.

Some Upsets
You Can Treat

Calves, just like people, sometimes have small upsets and sometimes have serious illnesses. The upsets may well be treated with home remedies, but the more serious illnesses require professional help.

Home remedies often completely clear up the upsets, but you should watch your calf carefully after even a slight illness — and don't hesitate to call your veterinarian if the calf does not improve or if it shows signs of worsening. Small upsets sometimes have a way of developing into serious illnesses, and you may have misdiagnosed the problem.

Here are some problems you probably can treat on your own:

Simple scours: Scouring is the most common of calf ailments and the first problem you're likely to face. Simple scours — that is scours (loose stool) without the complications of blood streaks, foaminess, off-color or bad odor — may be treated effectively by giving less feed, particularly milk. First cut back the amount by one-third, or by diluting the milk one-third with water. If the scours clear up, continue the smaller (or diluted) feeding.

If they do not clear up, you may administer calf scour boluses according to the package directions. Weigh or measure your calf before giving, for the dosage is determined by the size of the calf. Calf boluses are much easier to administer if they are first dipped in butter or margarine.

Bald spots: Missing patches of hair, especially around the ears, neck and rump area, may mean the calf is a host to red lice. Dusting with *rotenone* will bring quick relief.

Mild bloat: All healthy, well-fed calves are a little paunchy. Looked at from the front, immediately after eating, the calf even looks lop-sided, with a higher hump on its left side. This is normal. But a bloated calf looses this lop-sided paunch-iness and takes on a balloon-like, rounded look. Mild bloat is an accumulation of gas and may be treated as you would treat gas in a human — with baking soda.

The soda may be fed dry — sometimes a calf will lick it from the hand — or by dissolving two teaspoons of soda in two cups of water, emptying his water pail and leaving the soda water as his only liquid. Sometimes a calf that cannot be persuaded to take soda otherwise will take a soda solution readily from his regular nurser, even though he has been weaned.

Because bloat may become a chronic condition, the best cure is prevention. Bloat almost always is caused by overeat-ing, usually an unfamiliar grain or rich pasture. Clover and alfalfa pasture are especially liable to cause bloat if the calf eats too much of them when they are wet from rain, frost or dew. To prevent such overeating, always allow the calf an hour in the morning to eat his grain and hay before you turn him out to pasture. This also gives time for the sun to dry the grass.

Other home remedies for bloat which may help are to keep the calf walking by means of a halter, or to administer one quart of raw linseed oil to which two ounces of turpentine have been added. You also may give the regular adult human dose of an antacid medicine such as Pepto Bismol.

Pinkeye: The watery, irritated redness of the eyes may be a contagious infection, and often is caused by flies. Symptoms begin with one or both eyes becoming watery, then red and sometimes mattered over. Treatment should be initiated immediately, because a calf may be blinded by a severe case. It can be prevented by vaccination or treated with an antibiotic pinkeye ointment or spray.

Since Pinkeye symptoms also may be caused by a deficiency of Vitamin A — and because any eye disease may be improved by the addition of Vitamin A to the diet — a calf should have free access to good pasture or plenty of bright green hay daily. Otherwise the diet should be supplemented with cod liver oil or Vitamin A-D and E powder especially marketed for livestock.

Head colds: Yes, a calf can have head colds just like people. He can catch a cold from people and can transmit cold germs to the people who care for him.

His symptoms will be the same as yours when you have a cold — runny nose, watery eyes, a cough and chills. Treat his cold just as you would that of any youngster, with extra warmth, good food, a lot of care and a little medication. A child's dose of antihistamine may take care of his sniffles, and a warm bran mash or a little honey and an egg mixed in with his milk ration may encourage his appetite.

For a cough, two home remedies for children's colds also work well with a young calf: A medicine-filled vaporizer, placed just outside his stall and directed toward him, or a good chest rubdown with camphorated oil topped by a turtle-neck sweater or sweatshirt.

Although the calf is as uncomfortable as you are with a cold, the condition is not serious unless he develops pneumonia. Watch especially for a change in his temperature.

The dosage for all home remedies must be regulated according to the weight of the calf, not the age — for calves of the same age may vary greatly in weight. At birth a Holstein calf often weighs three times as much as an Angus calf. Weigh the calf on the barn scales or estimate his weight by eye or with a weigh-tape. Then adjust the dosage according to label directions. For instance, a 60 pound calf would be given one aspirin for fever, or one tablespoon of Kaopectate for mild scours or one teaspoon of baking soda for an upset stomach.

When the dosage directions are given according to the age of the child, the following adjustments may be used:

A 30- to 50-pound calf would get the same dosage as a two- to three-year-old child.

A 50- to 70-pound calf would compare to a six- or seven-year-old child.

A 100-pound calf would be given an adult dose.

Small upsets in your calf's health can be treated as you would treat those same upsets in a child, and with the same cautions. If it is an upset you would treat at home for a child, try a home remedy for the calf. If it is an illness for which you would rush your child to a doctor, call the veterinarian in.

The trick is in knowing when it's a small upset, or when you should call for help. If you're like most of us, you'll be more than likely to over- than to under-react. When in doubt call your veterinarian and ask *him* if he should come. If you have a good relationship with a nearby veterinarian whom you have consulted on vaccinations, dehorning and routine care, he probably won't mind. Even if he charges you for the telephone consultation and there was nothing to worry about, you can consider the charge an investment in your education.

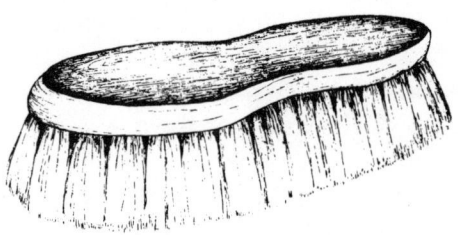

Other Illnesses Require a Veterinarian

Infectious scours: When scours are caused by bacterial infection rather than by overeating, it can be a serious condition which may cause the death of the animal in a short time. If the stool is a watery liquid which is forcibly ejected from the calf or if it is a green, foamy substance or is foul-smelling or blood streaked, give the calf electolyte solution in his nursing bottle and call the veterinarian. Do not try to treat infectious scours yourself.

Severe bloat: Bloat is the distention of the first two stomachs with gas. In severe cases of bloat the animal may die from suffocation if he is not helped immediately. An animal with acute bloat looks like a large balloon with four stiff legs. Often the only way to save such an animal is to puncture the paunch and release the pressure. Obtain help as quickly as possible if bloat is severe.

Calf diphtheria and pneumonia: A calf that refuses to eat, that appears listless and has difficulty breathing, may be suffering from calf diphtheria or pneumonia. Both are beyond the realm of home remedies. Call the veterinarian.

SYMPTOMS TO WATCH FOR

The following indicate illnesses that are beyond the skill of the inexperienced. If your calf should develop any of these symptoms, you should call a veterinarian immediately:

Foul-smelling breath, feces or hoofs: All are symptoms of a disease carried by the bacteria responsible for calf diphtheria and hoof rot. Hoof rot may be treated with iodine spray, while diphtheria requires the help of a veterinarian.

Noisy, labored breathing; A calf that is having difficulty breathing will thrust his head forward with his mouth open and his tongue hanging out. It is a sign of serious trouble, possibly pneumonia or calf diphtheria.

Skin sores: Sores on the skin may be a sign of lice or mite infestation, nutritional deficiency or abscesses.

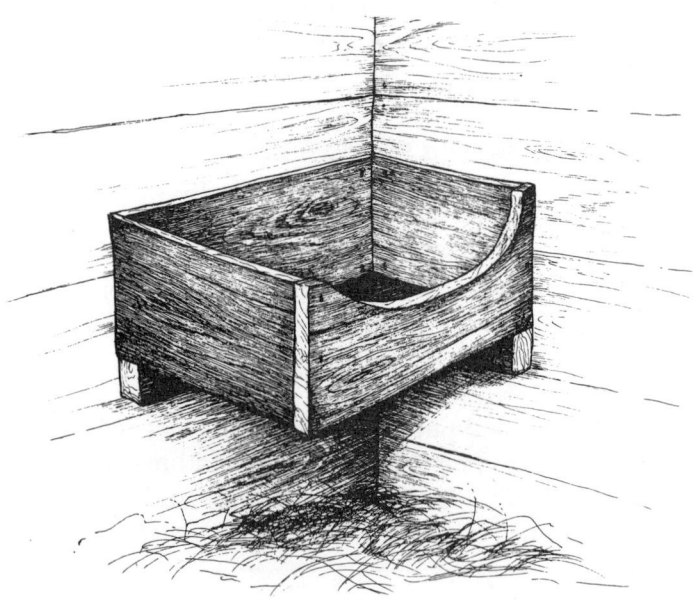

Unnatural positions; A sick calf stands with his back humped, his head down and his tail tucked between his legs, or he may lie on his side, with his head and legs stretched out. Either of these positions is a signal help is needed.

Scours: Look for watery, foamy, off-color or blood streaked stools. Scouring caused by bacterial infection needs treatment with antibiotics.

Lack of appetite: The final — and most serious — symptom displayed by a nursing calf is a lack of enthusiasm for food. Except for a newborn calf learning to nurse from a bottle, a calf that refuses to eat should have prompt attention.

Keep a Record

Even if you have only one calf, keep a record of his progress. This may be as simple as a card tacked on the barn wall (outside the calf's reach) or a notebook you keep in the house.

On this record note the calf's birth date, sex, his progressive weight, amount and frequency of feedings, any medications given and his general condition from day to day. Every morning after you have fed the calf, jot down the day, the feeding and his attitude that day.

You don't need a complicated system, but such a record may be invaluable in case allergies or illnesses develop or when you come to your second calf.

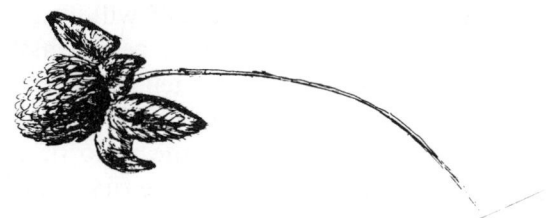

Fattening the Calf

How long you keep your calf will depend on your preference in beef, the size of your pasture and calf pens, and your supply of grain and hay.

If you prefer heavy, prime beef well-marbled with fat, you'll need to keep your calf at least two years. A two-year-old calf (yes, it's still called a calf at that age, since he isn't full-grown until he's about four years old) is still young enough to be tender but old enough to have acquired more flavor than younger beef. But the extra year of growth is costly, since it takes a year's supply of feed — about three tons of hay and one ton of grain — to increase the calf's weight 400 to 500 pounds.

A large, well-developed two-year-old calf will weigh between 1200 and 1500 pounds and will yield 750 to 900 pounds of beef. If you have pasture to see you through the summer, you may want to compromise by keeping your calf until he is 15 to 18 months of age. To cut grain costs, a spring calf may be kept on pasture for two summers and fed grain and hay only through one winter. A large, 18-month-old calf will weigh as much as 1000 to 1200 pounds and will dress out at 600 to 700 pounds.

At one year of age, a well-fed calf will weigh from 800 to 1000 pounds and is considered baby beef, which is preferred by some because it is exceptionally tender and, having less fat, lower in cholesterol than mature beef. The yearling calf is far more economical to raise, since the ratio of growth to the amount of grain fed is high. After the first year it takes more grain for every pound of growth. An 800 to 1000 pound calf will yield 470 to 500 pounds of beef, enough to feed a family of four for one year, assuming other meats also are used.

Calves which are grain-fed from birth produce a beef far superior to those which are raised on pasture only, then fattened in a barnlot for three months, the method most often used by commercial feeders. The costs are comparable since there is no need to overfeed grain just before butchering. The result is a nice, meaty calf with very little fat.

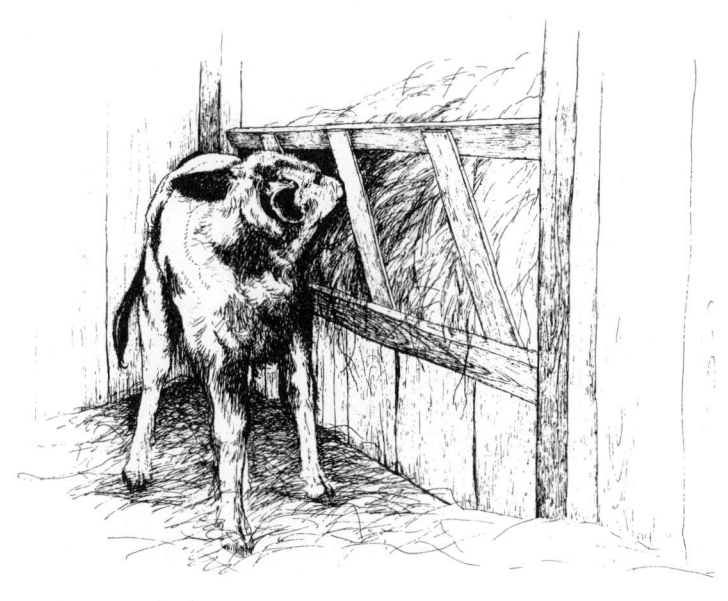

Butchering Time

When your calf is 18 to 20 months old and is sleek and looking well-fed, you may decide he is ready to butcher. After that age, he requires a great deal more feed to maintain condition and weight, and the ratio of gain to the amount of grain fed drops considerably. It also is best to butcher an animal when he is still young and tender. The best time is in the fall, when the calf is at the peak of condition from eating all that lush summer pasturage and before you must feed him expensive hay.

Unless you have a considerable experience in butchering, this is a job for a professional, usually a man in your area who advertises that he does custom butchering. All that is required is for you to transport the calf to his plant at a given time. For a reasonable fee — usually $10 plus the hide for killing, and a per-pound price for cutting, wrapping and quick freezing — he will have the meat ready for your home freezer in ten days to two weeks.

But good butchers are much in demand, so it is a good idea to call the one you have in mind at least six months in advance. Most are scheduled from three to six months ahead. At that time, you might also ask if transportation is available. Some butchers will arrange to pick up the animal at your barn for an additional fee.

"I don't see how you'll ever be able to eat that little brown-eyed baby after you raise him." You'll hear this — maybe from some members of your family — or you may even have said it yourself. But if you or any member of your family are concerned about whether or not you'll want to butcher the calf after it's raised, you should talk it over before you decide to raise one.

Remember that the little brown-eyed baby will no longer be a pet by the time he is 18 months old and weighs 1000 pounds. By then — especially if he is a bull calf — he probably will no longer trust humans and, except at feeding time, will come nowhere near you.

There is a psychological benefit, too, in having the butchering done away from home. There may be a moment of trauma the day the calf is sent away, but the packages of processed beef that are brought home are not easily associated with the animal. Many families buy another small calf just before the older calf is sent to the butcher. And many people refuse to give a name to any animal they intend later to butcher on the theory that the name gives it a personality.

But if members of the family — especially children — still object to the idea of butchering an animal, it may be a good idea to explain that livestock which are raised for food are the same as vegetables in the garden.

Your Beef on the Table

The accompanying chart shows the wholesale cuts of beef (inset) surrounded by the retail cuts, these expressed in their more familiar "butcher shop" names. Note also the suggestions for cooking and serving.

Although these are the most widely accepted cuts of beef, remember that any cut is satisfactory if it makes the most of the meat's tenderness and flavor. Some cuts may vary from the illustration according to the customs of your area, the style of the butcher and — in the case of custom butchering — the preferences of the consumer.

All cuts of lean beef have the same nutritional value, and when cooked correctly have the same good taste. But different cuts of beef vary in tenderness, so the cooking method should be determined by the cut's degree of tenderness.

For cooking with dry heat (roasting, broiling and pan-broiling) use tender cuts with small amounts of connective tissue — the ribs, loin and sirloin cuts, or ground beef.

For cooking with moist heat (braising, stewing and making soup) use the less-tender cuts, which are more economical if you are buying, and yet are equal in food value and flavor.

All cuts of beef may be made equally tender if you select the correct method of cooking or by grinding, pounding or marinating tougher cuts. Grinding or pounding will cut up or break down the connective tissue, while marinating (usually soaking the meat in some form of vinegar or tomato juice) will soften it.

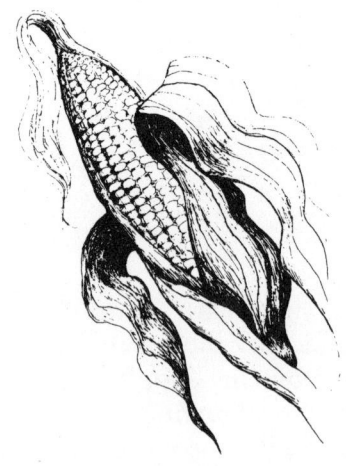

Beef Chart

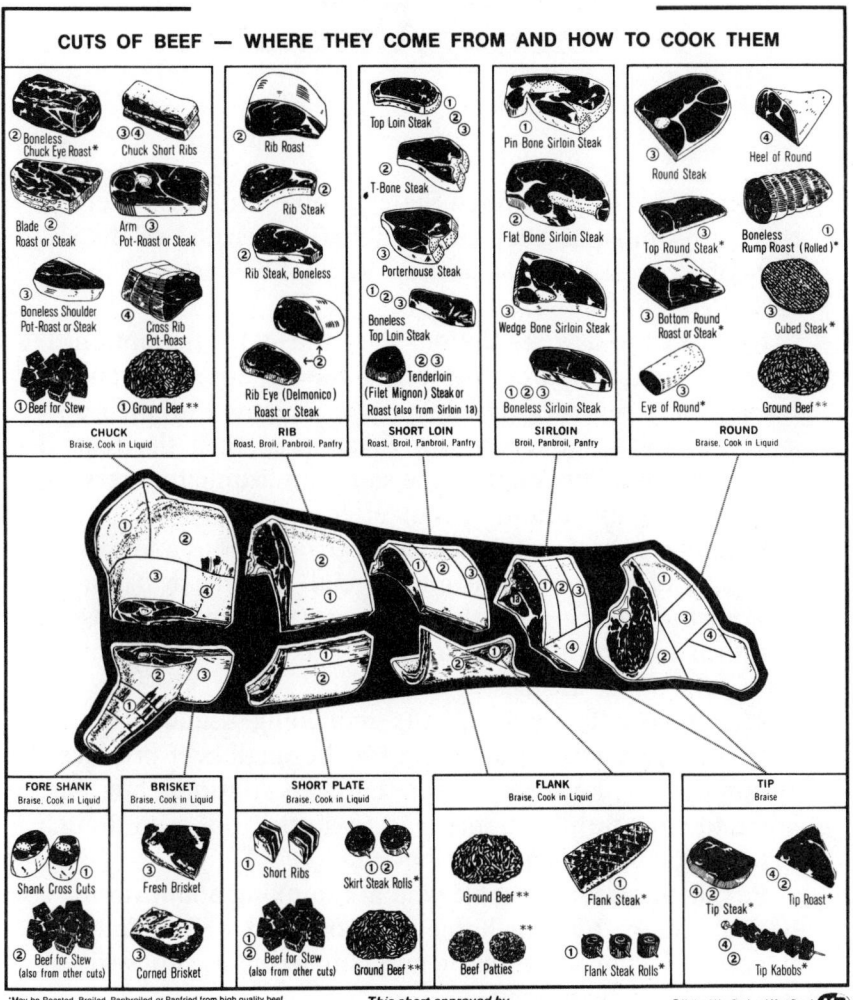

CUTS OF BEEF — WHERE THEY COME FROM AND HOW TO COOK THEM

CHUCK
Braise, Cook in Liquid

- ② Boneless Chuck Eye Roast*
- ③④ Chuck Short Ribs
- Blade ② Roast or Steak
- Arm ③ Pot-Roast or Steak
- ③ Boneless Shoulder Pot-Roast or Steak
- ④ Cross Rib Pot-Roast
- ① Beef for Stew
- ① Ground Beef**

RIB
Roast, Broil, Panbroil, Panfry

- ② Rib Roast
- ② Rib Steak
- ② Rib Steak, Boneless
- ←② Rib Eye (Delmonico) Roast or Steak

SHORT LOIN
Roast, Broil, Panbroil, Panfry

- ①②③ Top Loin Steak
- ② T-Bone Steak
- ③ Porterhouse Steak
- ①②③ Boneless Top Loin Steak
- ②③ Tenderloin (Filet Mignon) Steak or Roast (also from Sirloin 1a)

SIRLOIN
Broil, Panbroil, Panfry

- ① Pin Bone Sirloin Steak
- ② Flat Bone Sirloin Steak
- ③ Wedge Bone Sirloin Steak
- ①②③ Boneless Sirloin Steak

ROUND
Braise, Cook in Liquid

- ③ Round Steak
- ④ Heel of Round
- ③ Top Round Steak*
- ① Boneless Rump Roast (Rolled)*
- ③ Bottom Round Roast or Steak*
- ③ Cubed Steak*
- ③ Eye of Round*
- ① Ground Beef**

FORE SHANK
Braise, Cook in Liquid

- ① Shank Cross Cuts
- ② Beef for Stew (also from other cuts)

BRISKET
Braise, Cook in Liquid

- ③ Fresh Brisket
- ③ Corned Brisket

SHORT PLATE
Braise, Cook in Liquid

- ① Short Ribs
- ①② Skirt Steak Rolls*
- ①② Beef for Stew (also from other cuts)
- ① Ground Beef**

FLANK
Braise, Cook in Liquid

- ** Ground Beef**
- ① Flank Steak*
- ** Beef Patties
- ① Flank Steak Rolls*

TIP
Braise

- ④② Tip Steak*
- ④② Tip Roast*
- ④② Tip Kabobs*

*May be Roasted, Broiled, Panbroiled or Panfried from high quality beef.
**May be Roasted, (Baked), Broiled, Panbroiled or Panfried.

This chart approved by
National Live Stock and Meat Board

© National Live Stock and Meat Board

Butchering Alternatives

In some parts of the United States people who raise beef for themselves must do their own butchering because of the impact of Federal Meat Inspection Regulations enacted in the early 1970s.

In effect the new regulations gave the states the option to set their own standards (subject to federal approval) and to inspect and license local slaughterhouse plants with their own staffs. If the states chose *not* to do this, then the federal standards (and licensing) — the same applicable to interstate meat packing operations — took effect.

Federal standards are based on large operations and call for extensive plant equipment and special staffing. Most small custom butchering operations, therefore, have found it impractical to conform, and in these "federal" states usually have gone out of business.

The large commercial plants remaining usually are not geared to do custom butchering for the small beef producer. In some states, however, custom butchers continue, but must come to your farm or homestead to do the job, even though here the facilities usually are limited.

For these reasons, people who are thinking about raising a beef animal or two for home use would do well to find out in advance what slaughtering and butchering facilities will be available to them nearby.

If your state does not appear in this list, write to the meat inspection service of your state agriculture department for their list of state-licensed custom and commercial slaughter plants.

The "federal" states, where custom work may *not* be available, are:

Colorado	Nevada
Connecticut	New Jersey
Kentucky	New York
Massachusetts	North Dakota
Minnesota	Oregon
Missouri	Pennsylvania
Montana	Tennessee
Nebraska	Washington

Because of this possible problem in having your beef animal finished off, we present the following directions for doing your own slaughtering, cutting and processing of beef. This reprint of the often-used USDA Farmers Bulletin No. 2209 is perhaps the best and clearest guide available on the subject.

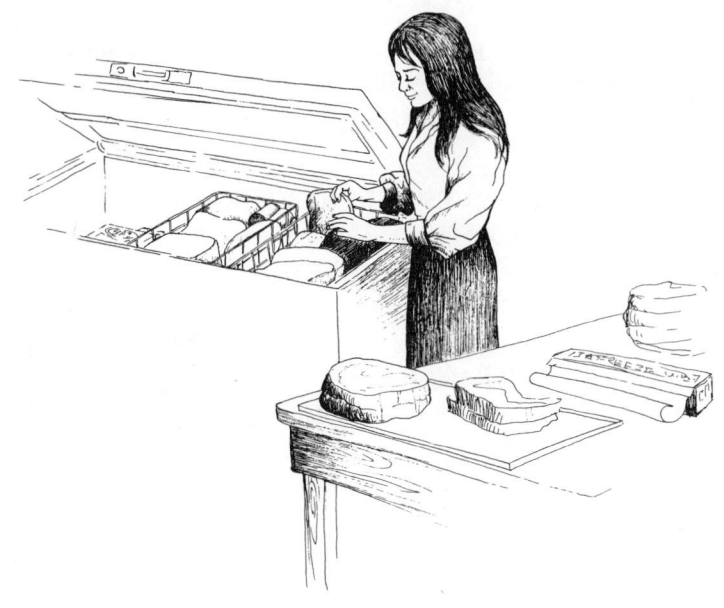

Further Reading

If you're involved in raising animals for food or profit, you will find many Garden Way books that will be helpful and instructive.

Here are some of them:

RAISING RABBITS THE MODERN WAY, by Robert Bennett. 156 pp., quality paperback, $4.95. Everything for the home and semi-commercial producer.

RAISING POULTRY THE MODERN WAY, by Leonard Mercia. 240 pp., quality paperback, $5.95. Outstanding in this field.

THE CANNING, FREEZING, CURING & SMOKING OF MEAT, FISH & GAME, by Wilbur F. Eastman Jr. 220 pp., quality paperback, $5.95; hardback, $8.95. Authoritative, easy-to-follow directions.

KEEPING THE HARVEST: HOME STORAGE OF VEGETABLES AND FRUITS, by Nancy Thurber and Gretchen Mead. 208 pp., quality paperback, $5.95; hardback, $8.95. Buy this one, and forget the other food storage books.

DOWN-TO-EARTH VEGETABLE GARDENING KNOW-HOW, featuring Dick Raymond. 160 pp., 8½ X 11", quality paperback, $5.95. A treasury of vegetable gardening information.

THE FAMILY COW, by Dirk van Loon. 270 pp., quality paperback, $5.95. Invaluable for the owner of a single cow or small herd. All of the answers are here, including what you should know if you are thinking of buying a cow and need advice. We recommend this highly.

RAISING SHEEP THE MODERN WAY, by Paula Simmons, 220 pp., quality paperback, $5.95. From breeding sheep to marketing them. Concise explanations for the beginner or veteran. It's packed with facts and advice on all stages of sheep-raising, from one who has learned by doing.

RAISING MILK GOATS THE MODERN WAY, by Jerry Belanger, editor of Countryside & Small Stock Journal. 152 pp., quality paperback, $4.95. Belanger knew the problems goat owners faced, the questions they wanted answered. This book gives the answers in down-to-earth, easy-to-understand terms.

These books are available at your bookstore, or may be ordered directly from Garden Way Publishing, Dept. RC, Charlotte, Vermont 05445. If order is less than $10, please add 75¢ postage and handling.

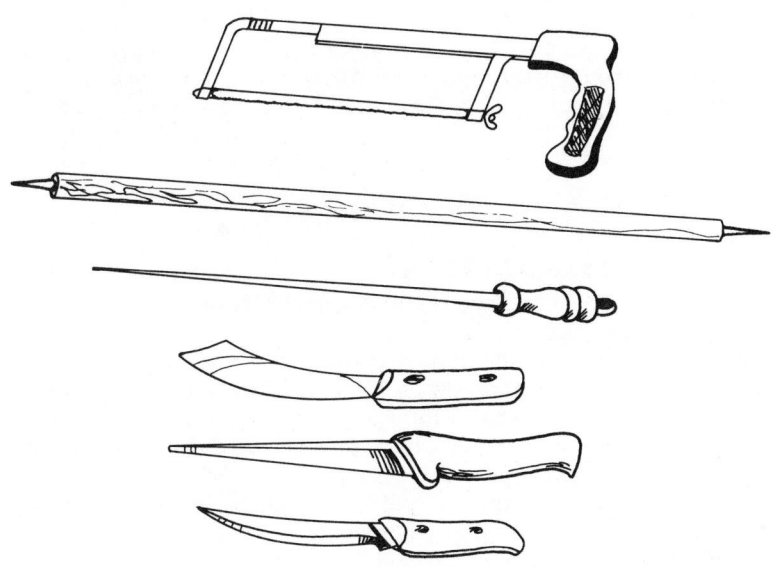

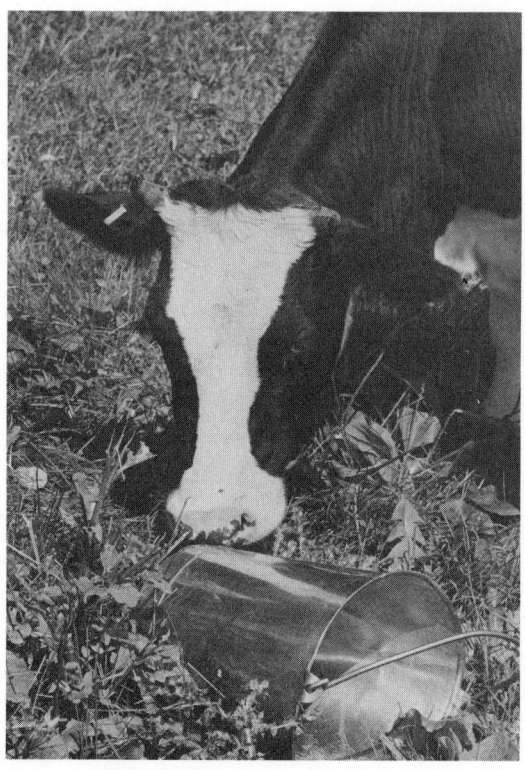

Success in preparing meat depends on strict attention to the methods used None of the details of these methods is difficult, but all are important.

PRECAUTIONS

Do not slaughter beef animals that have received an additive of diethylstilbestrol in their ration unless the additive has been withdrawn at least 48 hours prior to slaughter.

To control flies and other insects at the time of slaughtering, chilling, cutting, and processing, apply the proper insecticide. Use a product specifically labeled for this purpose or for use in dairy or milk-processing rooms. Follow instructions on the product label, observing all the precautions listed. Be sure to cover all equipment and working surfaces with a drop cloth before spraying. After you have sprayed, and before beginning slaughtering, chilling, cutting, and processing, thoroughly wash the equipment, tables, and floors with plenty of hot water and soap or detergent.

SLAUGHTERING, CUTTING AND PROCESSING BEEF ON THE FARM

By Richard L. Hiner, food products technologist, Animal Husbandry
Research Division, Agricultural Research Service

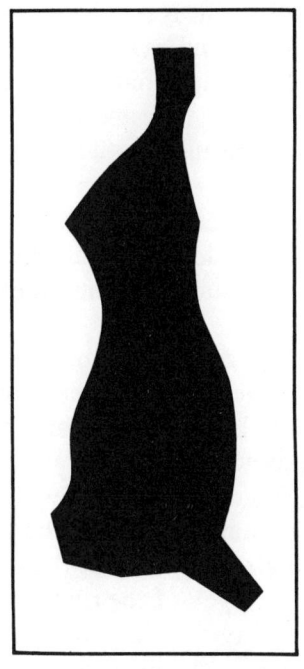 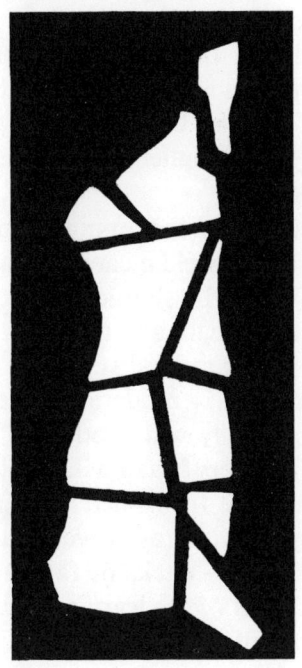

Farmers Bulletin No. 2209
U. S. DEPARTMENT OF AGRICULTURE

Selecting Animal for Slaughter

You should consider several factors before slaughtering and preparing a beef carcass for home consumption. The most important considerations are the breeding, feeding, management and age of the animal and method of handling the meat.

If at all possible, select for slaughter an animal representing one of the beef breeds. The reason for this is that beef animals are thicker fleshed, fatten more readily, and have more fat over the lean muscles with considerably less internal or waste fats than do dairy breeds. A well-finished beef-type animal will generally dress higher and will cut out more and meatier roasts and steaks.

Feeding of the animal is important because a well-finished animal will yield a carcass that has a moderately thick covering of fat over the shoulders, back, and round, without an excess of internal caul and ruffle fat.

A young animal such as a yearling or a 2-year-old steer or heifer that is moderately well finished and has made good gains usually will produce a carcass having tender and more desirable meat than will an older, more mature animal.

The meat from such an animal, in good condition, will ordinarily be moderately well marbled; that is, there will be small visible white flecks of fat intermingled throughout the cross-section cut of the lean, especially the "eye" of the rib and loin. There will be a rather smooth, even layer of fat over the outside of the dressed carcass. Such an animal will, as a rule, have lean meat that is bright cherry red.

An animal that has been fattened on grass and grain may

have slightly yellow fat and be slightly softer in the firmness of the lean. However, this should not detract from the quality of the beef carcass, as yellow color indicates additional carotene, an essential nutritive property.

Proper handling of the dressed beef carcass and cuts is important in insuring quality. The first indication of proper handling is appearance, always a psychological factor and sometimes associated with characteristics of real importance. For example, a change in appearance that may occur is that caused by holding the fresh carcass or cuts at too high a temperature. The exposed lean will be dark and covered with slimy growth, as contrasted to that held for aging at 33° to 35° F. for extended periods to ripen. The latter will be covered with a dry-appearing mold that can be easily removed by trimming. Improper chilling will result in difficulty of cutting and preparing smooth, firm cuts. It must be remembered that one cannot improve the quality of the meat, but one can easily spoil an otherwise high-quality beef carcass.

Care and Handling of Animal Before Slaughter

Proper care of an animal before slaughter is important in obtaining more high-quality meat from your finished animal.

Pen the animal by itself the day before slaughtering.

Keep the animal off feed 24 hours before slaughtering, but provide access to water at all times.

Running, exciting, or whipping the animal may cause a temporary fever. If the animal is killed in this condition, the meat is likely to be bloody and fiery in color, fail to bleed properly,

and have numerous bruised areas that are a complete and un-
necessary loss.

Slaughtering

EQUIPMENT

Elaborate and expensive equipment is unnecessary but certain
tools are essential. The following equipment is recommended:

- Stunning hammer (mechanical) or .22 caliber rifle.
- 6-inch skinning knife.
- Block and tackle or chain hoist.
- Beef spreader (a doubletree will do).
- Cleaver.
- 28-inch meat saw with heavy blade.
- Pritch pole about 2½ feet long.
- 12-inch steel.
- Good oil or water stone.
- 12-inch straight-blade steak knife.
- 2½-foot length of log chain with a large ring at one end.
- Ample cold water and clean cloths.
- Bucket.

STUNNING

Kill the beef animal as humanely as possible and in a way that
will insure thorough drainage of blood. Fasten the animal's
head securely in a position that will enable you to stun it with
one sharp blow with a mechanical stunner or by shooting. The

proper place to strike is at the intersection of two imaginary lines extending from the right horn or edge of poll to the left eye and from the left horn or edge of poll to the right eye (fig. 1). A sharp blow at this point will immobilize the animal for several minutes. Stunning an animal is preferable to shooting it. After shooting, complete and efficient bleeding is not probable, and the results are bloody cuts, hastened spoilage, and unsightly roasts and steaks.

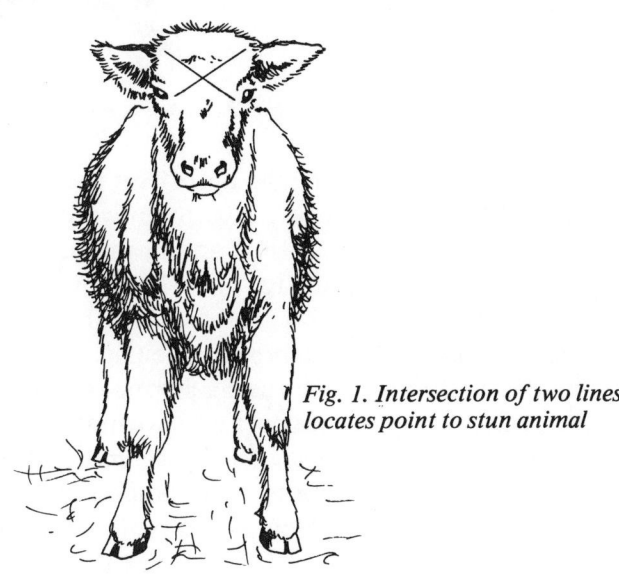

Fig. 1. Intersection of two lines locates point to stun animal

BLEEDING

As soon as the animal is down, draw a chain securely around the animal's hind legs and hoist it from the ground. The head of the animal should clear the floor by 18 to 24 inches. Grasp the left foreleg of the animal with your left hand and bend the leg back slightly. With the sharp skinning knife in your right hand, make an incision through the hide a little to the right of the middle of the dewlap. Extend the incision from the crease in front of the forelegs to the jawbone in the head.

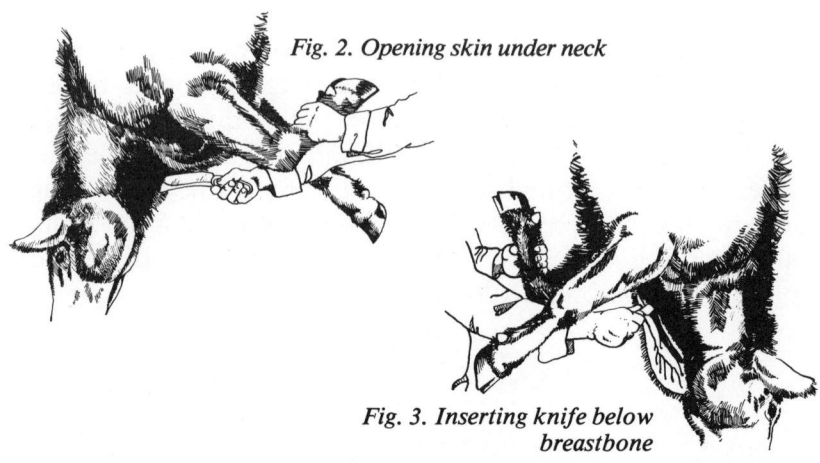

Fig. 2. Opening skin under neck

Fig. 3. Inserting knife below breastbone

The next step is to turn the knife over (sharp edge up) and, while holding the knife at a slightly upward angle, insert the point into the prepared incision and push it upward toward the point of the breastbone (fig. 2). When you reach the breastbone, follow downward with the point of the knife until the blade just slips under the breastbone (fig. 3) and between the first ribs. Cut straight to the backbone on either side of the gullet, then turn the knife over and downward. This will sever the carotid arteries as they fork just under the point of the breastbone. Take care not to stick too deeply and too far back into the chest cavity, which would permit the blood to accumulate in the chest cavity. Do not stick the heart; let it pump out the blood as long as possible. Make bleeding more complete by pumping the forelegs up and down a few times.

SKINNING

Skin out the forelegs and head and remove them as soon as bleeding has been completed. Remove forelegs by first cutting across the leg between the sole of the foot and the dewclaws, thus severing the tendon and releasing the tension of the leg. Split the skin over the back of the forelegs from the cut to a point 4 or 5 inches above the knee. Skin around the knees and shins and unjoint at the square joint (fig. 4).

Skin out the head by cutting back of the poll, then open the hide from poll to nostril. Skin across the head and over the right side, then over the left side to the jaws (fig. 5).

Remove the head by holding the loosened hide up in the left hand and cutting across the neck on a line just above the poll or through the Atlas joint (fig. 6).

Immediately on severing the head, thoroughly wash it with cold water to remove any regurgitated food and blood. Remove the tongue by an incision just inside each jaw, cutting forward to the point where they join; cut through the cartilage at the end of the bones that are located at the tongue's base; next, pull the tongue out and complete removal (fig. 7). Remove cheek meat from each side of the jawbone by cutting close to the bone and down to the rise of the bone just over each eye. Now, turn over the head and split with a cleaver or saw to remove the brains. Place the tongue and cheek meat in a bucket of cold water and allow to chill.

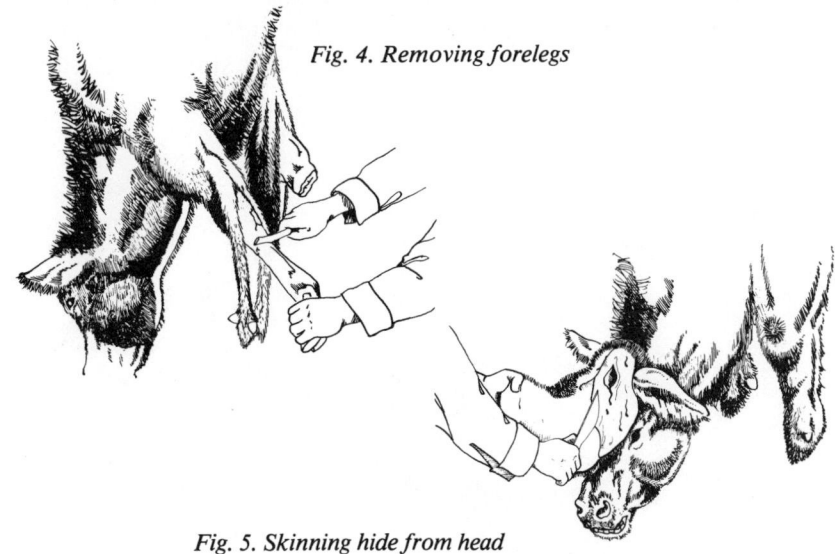

Fig. 4. Removing forelegs

Fig. 5. Skinning hide from head

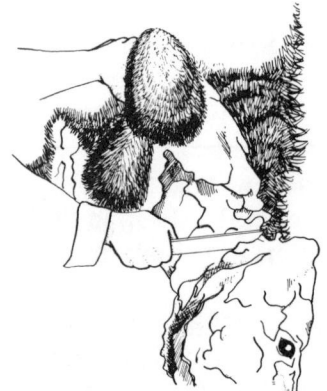

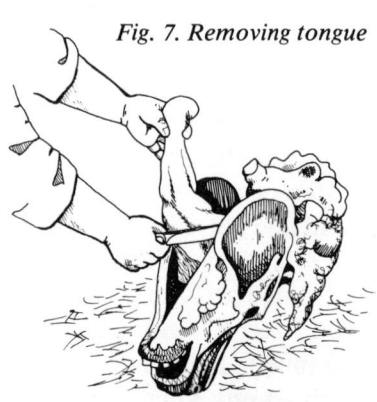

Fig. 7. Removing tongue

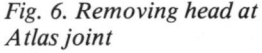

Fig. 6. Removing head at
Atlas joint

Lower the carcass to the floor, roll it on its back, and prop it in place with a pritch pole (fig. 8). Remove the hind legs by cutting across the tendons between the sole of the foot and the dewclaws, to permit the leg to relax. Split the skin from the dewclaws to the hock and over the rear of the thigh to a point about 6 inches below the hock joint (figs. 9 and 10). Remove the leg bone by cutting around the lowest joint of the hock (fig. 11). You can easily locate this joint with a knife. After marking the joint with a knife, give the leg a quick sideward push, and it will break apart.

Fig. 8. Carcass propped in
position with a pritch pole

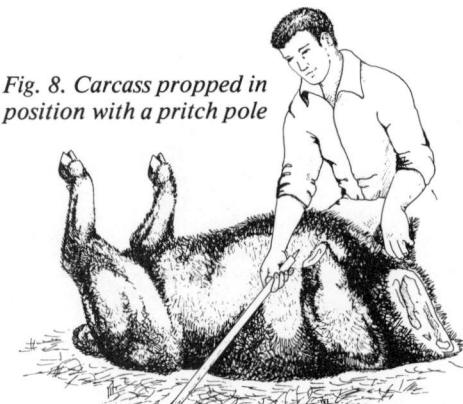

Fig. 9. Opening skin on hind leg

Fig. 10. Leg skinned and knife inserted to divide tendons

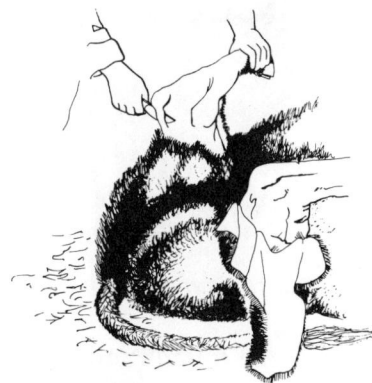

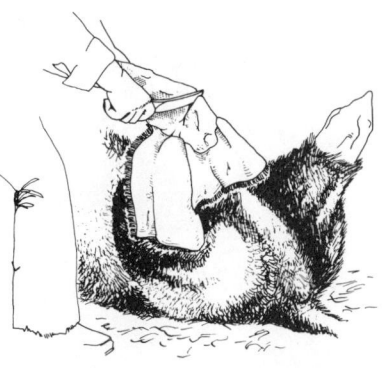

Fig. 11. Removing shank at lower hock joint

OPENING CARCASS AND SIDING

As the next step, split the skin from the point in front of the breastbone to the rump. You can do this by first placing the knife in the opening in the neck made for bleeding the animal and drawing it straight back over the brisket and just past the last rib, cutting through the hide and meat over the breastbone (fig. 12).

Now cut the hide at the midpoint between the hind legs, exposing a round muscle. Beginning at the last rib, cut through the hide and abdominal wall and continue the cut back to the opening between the hind legs, exposing the paunch. Make this cut carefully to avoid puncturing the paunch or intestines. It is a good plan to grasp the skin and flesh with the left hand. Then with your right hand, hold the knife blade with point up inside the abdominal cavity and push the knife in a straight line to the opening between the hind legs (fig. 13).

Split the skin on the inside of the thighs as shown in figure 14, beginning just back of the scrotum or udder, and cutting upward to the split made in removing the hind shank. Turn the knife down flat, with the edge pointed outward and a little upward to avoid cutting the flesh. Skin the inside of the thighs

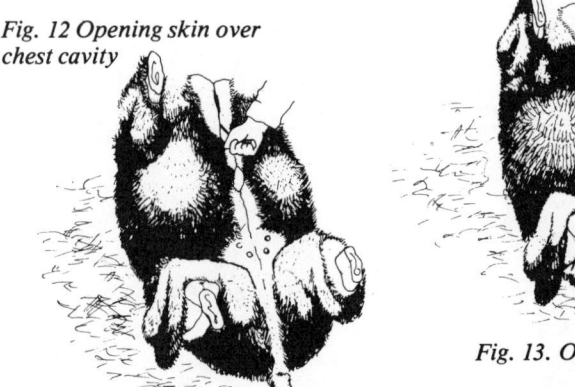

Fig. 12 Opening skin over chest cavity

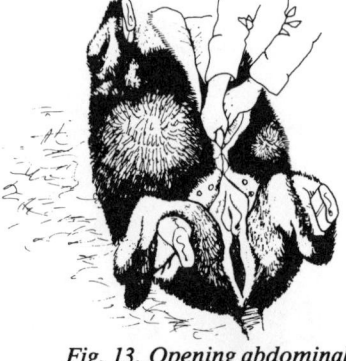

Fig. 13. Opening abdominal cavity

well down, but do not skin the outside of the rounds until the carcass has been raised. Skin the forelegs in similar manner.

The next and most important part of skinning is known as "siding." The knife must be sharp and have a smooth, keen edge, and must be steeled frequently. Keep a separate knife for siding only. Begin the siding by running the knife under the skin that has been cut over the abdomen. Grasp this loosened skin in the left hand and pull it up and outward. Grasping the knife as shown in figure 15, place the knife firmly against the hide, with the blade turned slightly outward to avoid cutting the flat muscles covering the abdomen and side. With sweeping strokes of the knife, continue siding until you cannot conveniently cut down further.

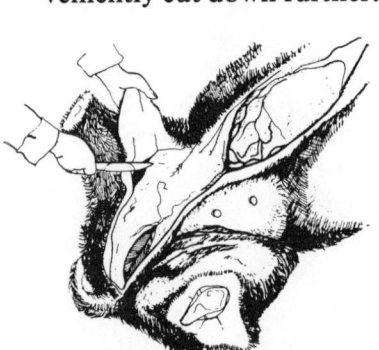

Fig. 14. Skinning thigh

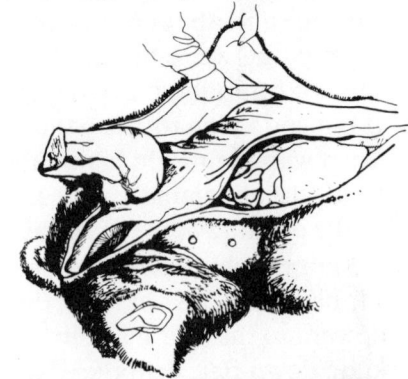

Fig. 15. Siding—note hide being stretched and angle of knife blade

Remove skin in like manner over the shoulders and round as shown in figure 16. Leave the "fell," or thin membrane that lies between the meat and skin, on the carcass. This membrane protects the meat from drying too rapidly and from attack by molds.

HOISTING

Prepare the carcass for hoisting by first sawing through the breastbone (fig. 17) and completing the separation of the rounds and splitting or sawing the aitchbone (fig. 18). Locate the point at which the aitchbone, or pelvic arch, is cut by finding the middle "seam," a small bony projection that can be felt with the finger just under the front (forward side) of the pelvis. Next, insert the spreader between the large tendons that were separated earlier. Hoist the carcass with a hoist or block and tackle to a convenient working height to skin the rounds. Skin the rounds, being careful to leave the "fell" attached to the fat covering (fig. 19).

Next, cut the hide down the center of the tail to nearly the last joint. Cut joint, pull hide off, then disjoint the tail at its base (fig. 20). Wipe the hocks and rounds with a clean cloth dipped in warm water and wrung dry.

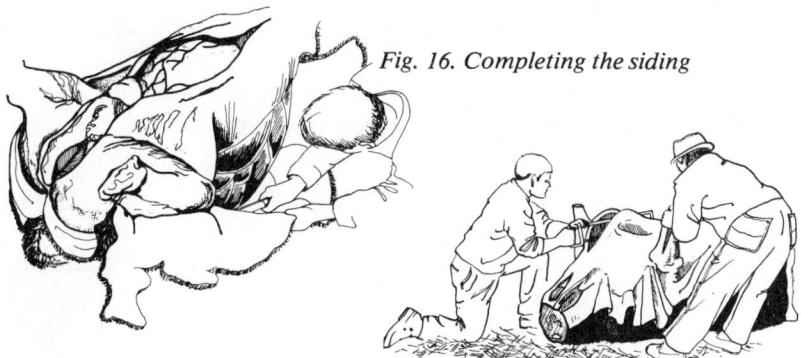

Fig. 16. Completing the siding

Fig. 17. Sawing breastbone

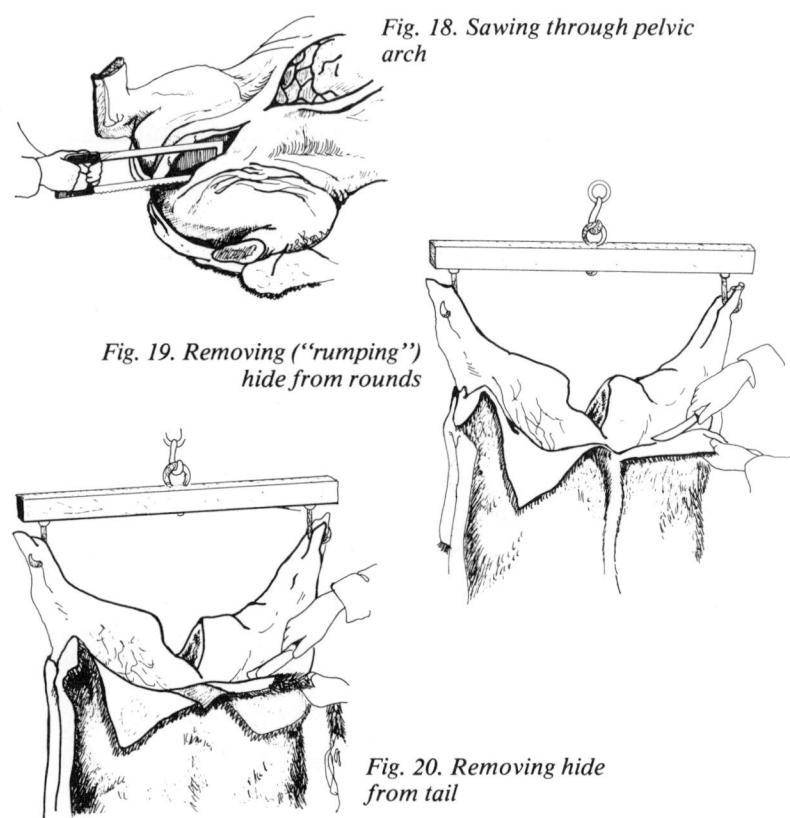

Fig. 18. Sawing through pelvic arch

Fig. 19. Removing ("rumping") hide from rounds

Fig. 20. Removing hide from tail

REMOVING VISCERA

Loosen the anus by cutting around it on the two sides and back, then loosening about 12 to 15 inches of the colon and allowing it to drop down over the paunch. Hoist the carcass until it clears the floor. Place a large container between the forelegs; with a knife, cut free the connective tissue that holds the intestines (fig. 21). Use care not to tear the kidney and bedfat. Pull down on the paunch to tear it loose from the carcass and allow it to fall into a container. As the paunch falls, be sure the liver is not attached to it. A small cut with a knife will free the liver and intestines (fig. 22). Insert a finger under the gall bladder and pull it off. Remove the liver.

Remove the heart and lungs by cutting out the diaphragm (the thin sheet of muscle and white connective tissue that separates them from the stomach and intestines). Allow 3 or 4 inches of the diaphragm to remain attached to the carcass. Grasp the loosened diaphragm and pull it outward and down, loosening the heart and lungs by cutting the large vessel (aorta) attached to the back bone. Remove heart, lungs, and gullet as one unit.

Fig. 21. Loosening the viscera

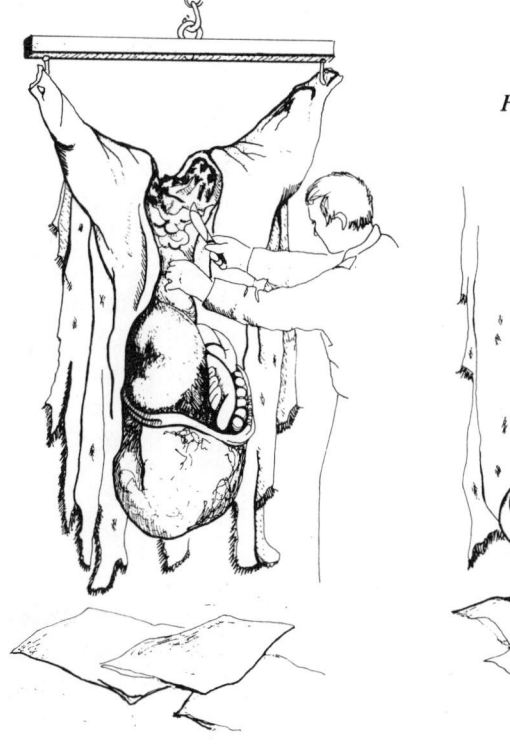

Fig. 22. Cutting viscera loose from liver

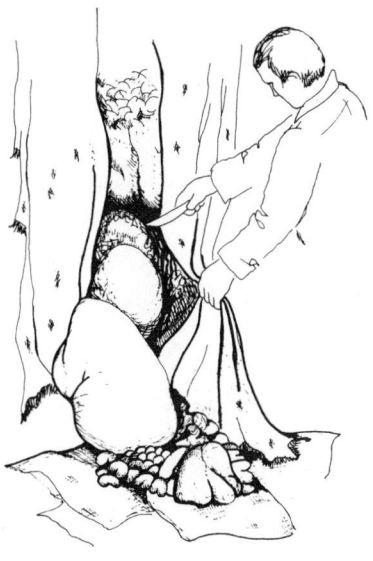

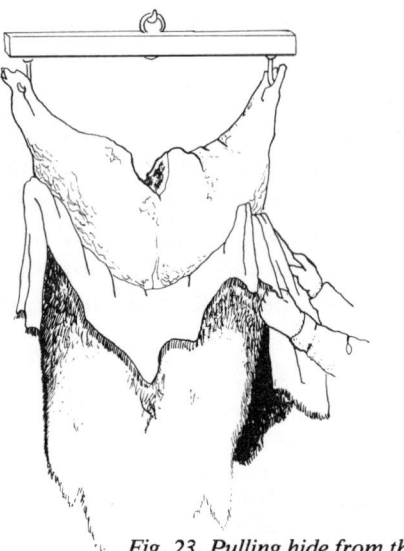

Fig. 23. Pulling hide from thigh

Lower the carcass until it just clears the floor, for convenience of skinning the hind quarters. Remove the hide by grasping the loose leg portions and pulling down (fig. 23). If the hide does not yield readily, loosen it by cutting a little with a knife, then pulling. You can pull the hide over the sides if it has been started properly. If these methods do not give satisfactory results, remove the hide with a knife, using the same procedure as in "siding." Continue removing the hide down over the shoulders, allowing the hide to remain attached over the neck.

SPLITTING THE CARCASS

Split the warm, dressed carcass into two halves. This allows for free circulation of air around the halves, thus a quicker chill. A dressed carcass is heavy and difficult to handle if it is not split. In splitting a beef carcass, start the split by first sawing through the sacral vertebrae from the inside (fig. 24). As soon as you have made the cut to the rise of the pelvic arch, you can do the sawing more satisfactorily from the back. Before starting to saw from the back, use a knife to mark the line you wish the saw to take. Make this cut over the top of the bony spinal process, which can be easily located with the fingers (fig. 25). Make the split down the center of the backbone and as far as the neck. As the backbone is split, hoist the dressed carcass for convenience sawing.

You are now ready to remove the hide from the forelegs and neck (fig. 26). You can split the neck and free the two halves. It is easier to split the neck with a sharp cleaver (fig. 27). Wash the carcass in cold water to remove all blood and dirt. Pump the forelegs up and down a few times to aid in draining blood from the forequarters. Trim loose and ragged pieces of meat.

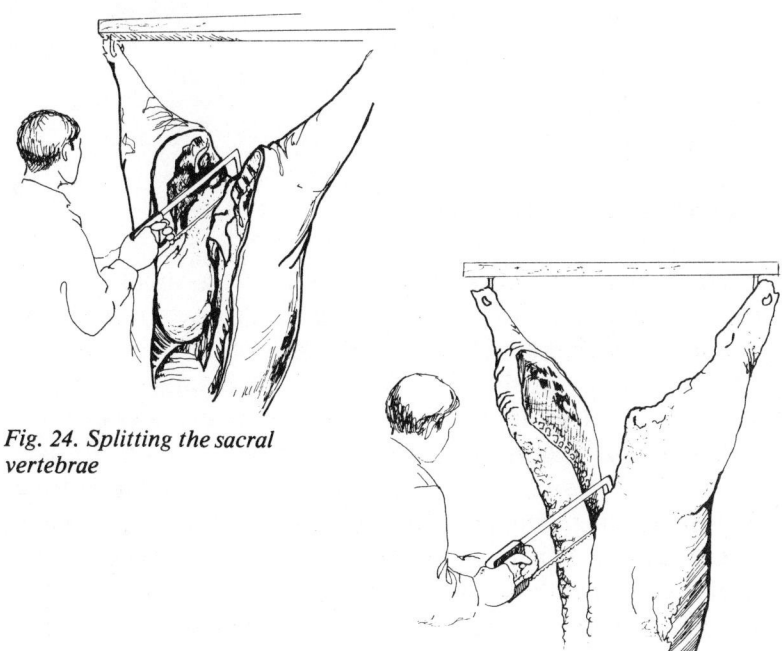

Fig. 24. Splitting the sacral vertebrae

Fig. 25. Splitting down the back

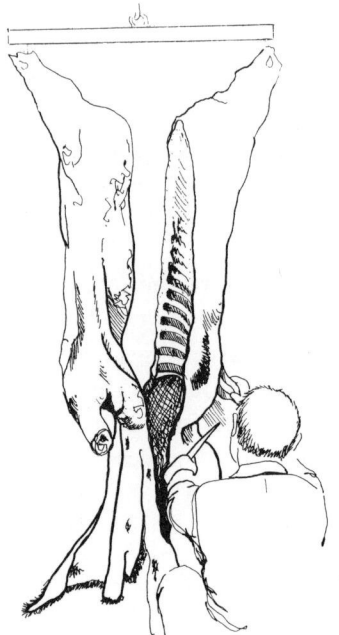

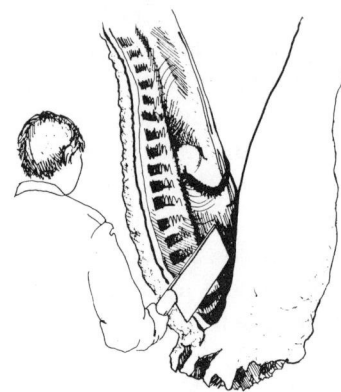

Fig. 27. Splitting neck with cleaver

Fig. 26. Removing hide from neck and forelegs

EXAMINING THE CARCASS

All the internal organs and the dressed carcass should be carefully examined at the time of slaughter for any abnormalities or conditions that might affect the fitness of the meat for food. The only person qualified to do this is a graduate veterinarian. Bruises, minor injuries, parasites in the organs, and enclosed abscesses, single tumors, and so on frequently are local conditions that can be easily removed. However, the presence of congestion or inflammation of the lungs, intestines, kidneys, inner surface of chest, or abdominal cavity and numerous yellowish or pearl-like growths scattered throughout the organs should be viewed seriously. Carcasses having such abnormalities should be examined by a graduate veterinarian and his opinion obtained as to the wholesomeness of the meat.

CARE OF THE INTERNAL ORGANS

As soon as you remove the liver, examine it for abscesses and other abnormalities and, if you find it clean, place it in a tub of cold water. Cut off the heart through the auricles and open it to remove any blood clots; then place it in a tub of cold water. As soon as you remove the tongue, scrape it free of all food and chill in cold water. Cut off the meat along the side of the jawbones and place in cold water to chill. After chilling for an hour or so, remove the liver, heart, tongue, tail, and cheek meat and hang up to drain and dry.

Separate the caul fat from the stomach with the hands. Remove or "run" the small intestines from the ruffle fat by pulling the intestines in one section with the left hand and cutting them free of the fat with a knife in the right hand. You can save the caul and ruffle, if not fouled in dressing, and use as tallow for soap.

The first and second stomachs are frequently used for making tripe. This is prepared by cutting off the two stomachs and emptying their contents by turning them inside out after slitting. Wash the stomachs thoroughly and rinse several times in clean, cold water, then hang up to drain.

CHILLING THE CARCASS

The tissues of many freshly slaughtered beef carcasses contain bacteria that can spoil the meat unless their growth is promptly checked. This is especially true of the thicker portions of the carcass, such as the rounds and shoulders.

Packers have practically solved the problem of bone sours by chilling the fresh, warm carcass to an internal temperature of less than 40° F. within 24 hours. The chilled carcass is held at 32° to 34° F. until cut.

On the farm, do slaughtering when the weather is most favorable. However, do not allow the freshly dressed carcass to freeze before chilling. When necessary to protect it from freezing, hang the carcass in a well-ventilated shed, or wrap it with a sheet. Wrapping not only will help protect against freezing, but will also help to smooth out the outer surface of the dressed carcass. Tightly draw the cloth around the carcass and securely fasten it with skewers.

It is often advantageous to allow chilled dressed beef carcasses to age several days before cutting. This aging allows the meat to pass through a period of rigor mortis, which requires 3 to 5 days. Additional aging of 10 to 15 days, if temperature conditions of 32° to 34 ° F. are favorable, will be beneficial in improving the tenderness of the meat. Chilled beef carcasses aged for this length of time should be well covered with fat and be protected from the weather, unless they are held in a cooler with controlled temperatures.

Suspend split beef carcasses to chill. Do not allow them to come in contact with each other. Free circulation of air around the dressed carcass is essential to proper chilling. If hot, dressed sides are allowed to touch, chilling is delayed and bone taint and spoilage will occur. The need for prompt and thorough chilling of warm carcasses cannot be overemphasized.

FREEZER PLANTS[1]

Most communities have access to local cold-storage as well as freezer locker plants with facilities to chill the carcass, prepare and freeze selected cuts, and age or store the fresh meat. Many plants have facilities for slaughtering cattle. If these facilities are not available, or if you wish to do your own slaughtering, you can bring the warm, dressed sides of beef immediately to the cold-storage plant and chill them. After chilling the carcass and aging it for the desired time, you should return to cut the beef and prepare it for the freezer or curing. In a cooperative cold-storage plant, nominal charges often can be obtained.

---

[1]For further information on freezing and storage, consult you county agricultural agent or write to the U.S. Department of Agriculture, Washington, D.C. 20250.

Cutting

CUTTING THE CARCASS

There is no one *best* method for cutting a beef carcass. The choice depends on how the beef is to be used. If it is to be sold, the cuts should conform to local preferences. If the meat is to be preserved by freezing, each piece should be of a size and character suitable for convenient cooking. The purpose of the method described here is to produce the maximum quantity of meat that can be preserved and stored.

QUARTERING OR "RIBBING"

Locate the last rib, or count up 12 ribs from the neck. Insert the knife blade between the twelfth and thirteenth rib at a point midway between the backbone and flank, marked *number 1* in figure 28. Following the angle of the rib, cut on a line parallel with the ribs to the backbone, marked *number 2* in figure 28. Turn knife around and cut toward the flank. As soon as the knife has cut through the cartilage at the end of the ribs, arch it downward until the cut is on the same level as that at the backbone marked *number 3* in figure 28, leaving 4 or 5 inches of the flank uncut to hold up the forequarter when the backbone has been sawed (fig. 29).

THE FOREQUARTER

At this point, remove the prime rib. Count up five ribs and insert knife between the fifth and sixth rib, (point *number 4,* fig.

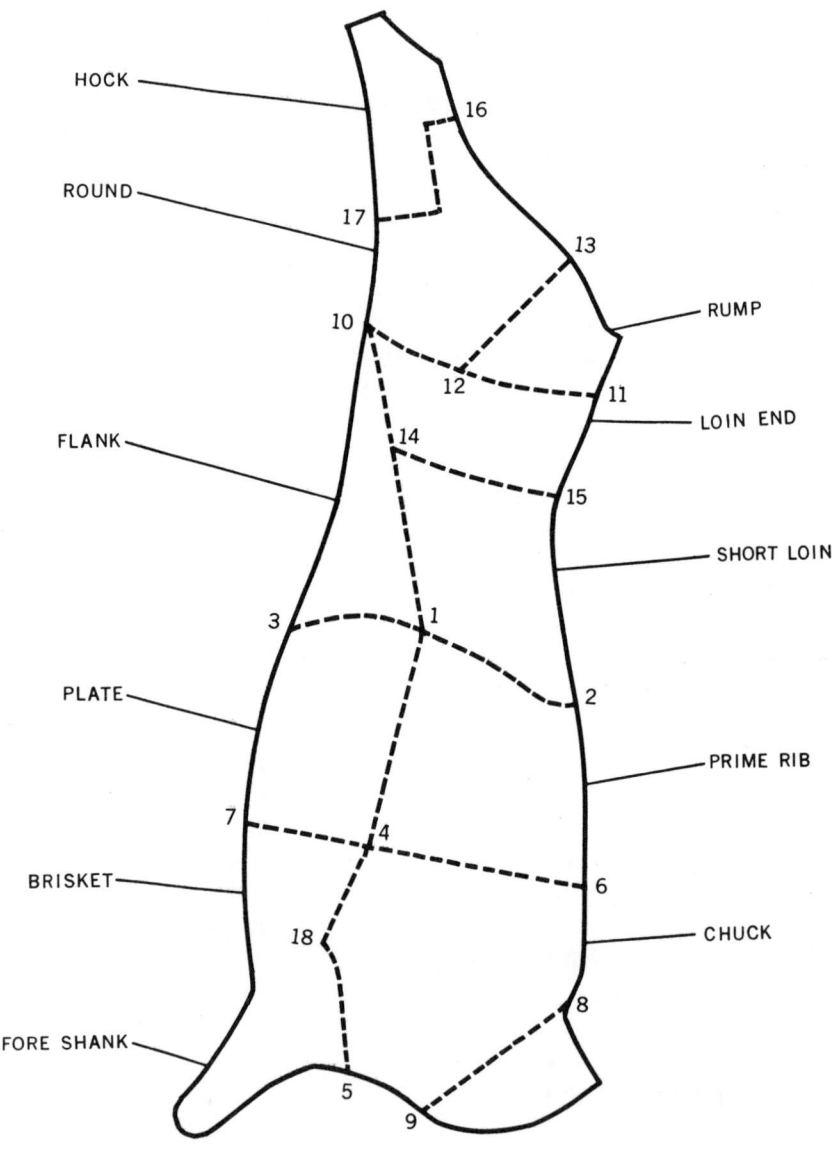

Fig. 28. Side of beef with primary cuts outlined and named

28) making a short cut (fig. 30). Mark a point that is about two-thirds of the distance between point *number 2* and the bottom or end of the cartilage (point *number 1,* fig. 28). From point *number 1,* cut on a line from *1* to *4* and across to *number 6* (fig. 28). With a hand meat saw, cut through the rib bones (*1* to *4*) and then the backbone at *number 6* (figs. 31 and 32).

Free the remaining forequarter by cutting the flank at point *number 3.* Place rattle on table, bone side down. Remove fore-shank by marking line *4* to *5* (fig. 28), and sawing across large bone (fig. 33). Now cut shank free. The cut across the humerus should be at right angles to the humerus and about 3 inches up from the joint (see point *A,* fig. 33). Cut through the meat to the ribs along line *4* to *5* (fig. 28). Saw along this line and remove plate and brisket (fig. 34). Remove neck by cutting on

Fig. 29. Separating carcass into fore and hind quarters

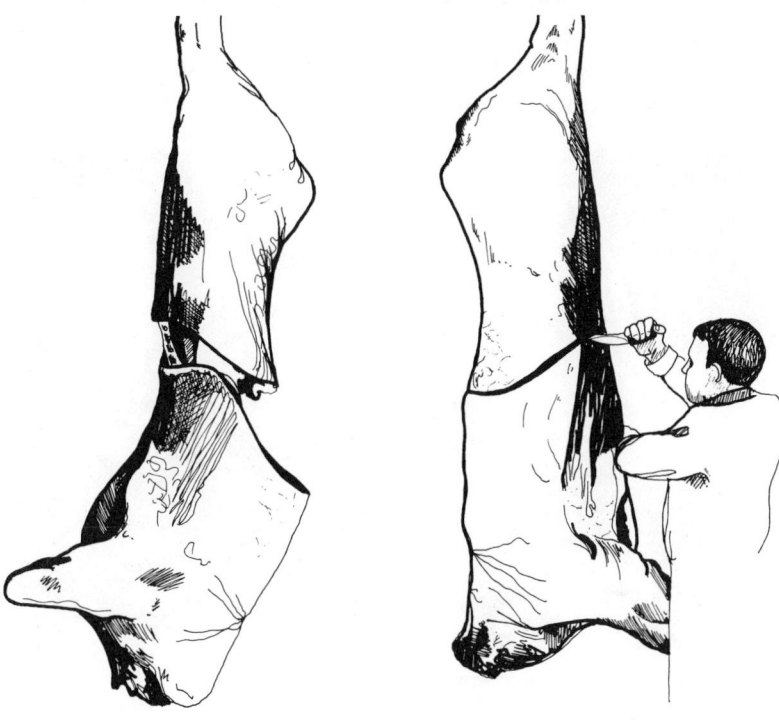

line *8* to *9* (fig. 28), marking it first with a knife and then sawing through the neck vertebrae (fig. 35).

You are now ready to divide the forequarter cuts into usable pieces. The square-cut chuck can be divided into pot roasts by first cutting a roast of the desired thickness over the fifth rib, then over the round bone, and so on. If you desire, you may remove several steaks first (fig. 36). Cut the foreshank into several small sections for boiling (fig. 37), or bone it and grind the meat as hamburger, and use the bone for soup. Divide the prime rib into several standing rib roasts, each consisting of one or more ribs (fig. 38). Strip the outer white fascia from the breast by first making a cut along the edge, then raising it with the fingers and stripping out (fig. 39).

You can divide this long breast cut into brisket and plate by separating it into two parts, line *4* to *7* in figure 28 (fig. 40). The brisket portion is useful as corned beef. Cut the plate in half, then into sections consisting of one to three ribs and use as short ribs (fig. 41). Bone the neck portion and use the meat as hamburger and the bone for soup.

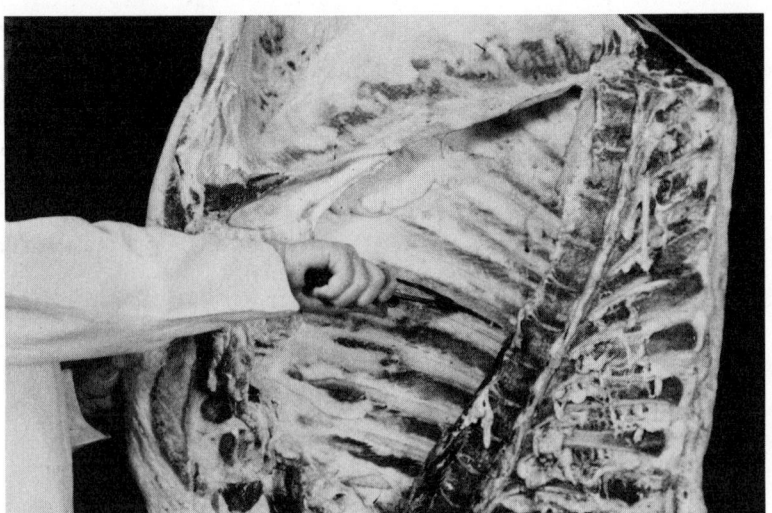

Fig. 30. Marking point to remove prime rib

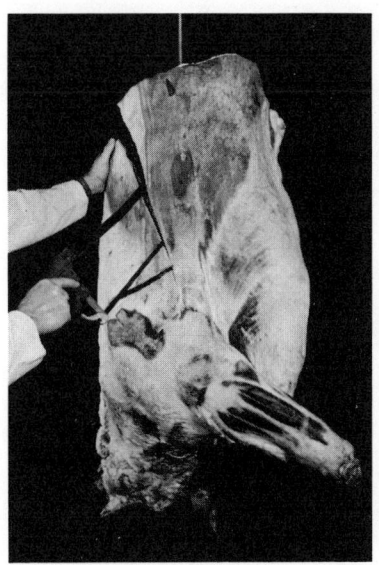

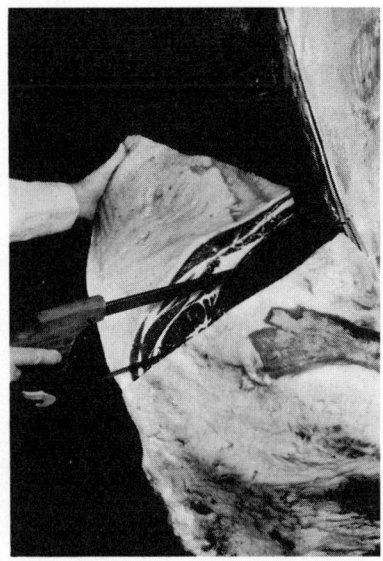

Fig. 31. Separating prime rib from plate

Fig. 32. Sawing prime rib from chuck

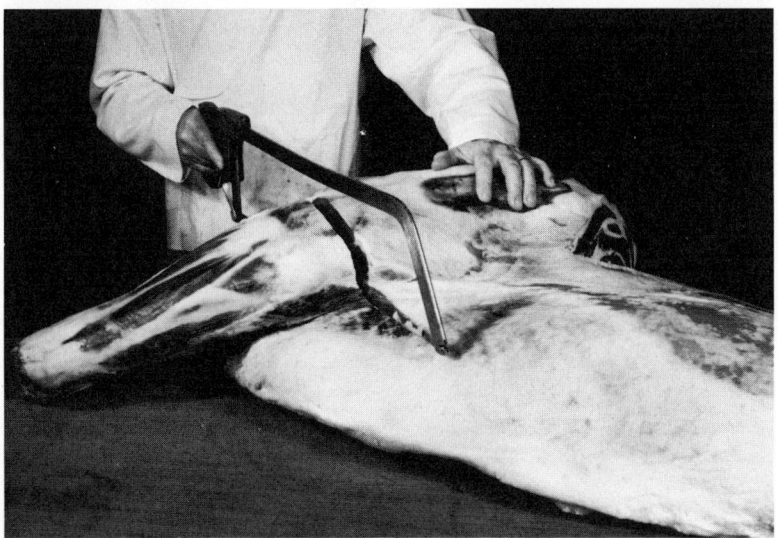

Fig. 33. Removing foreshank

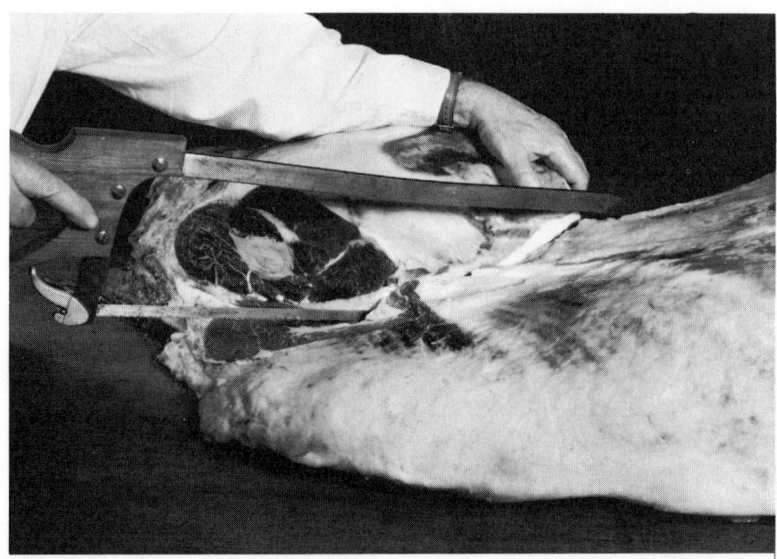

Fig. 34. Removing plate and brisket from chuck

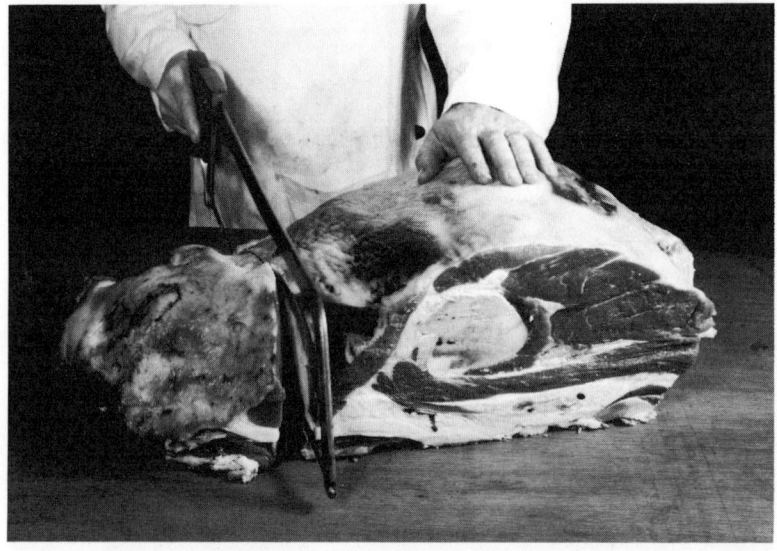

Fig. 35. Removing neck

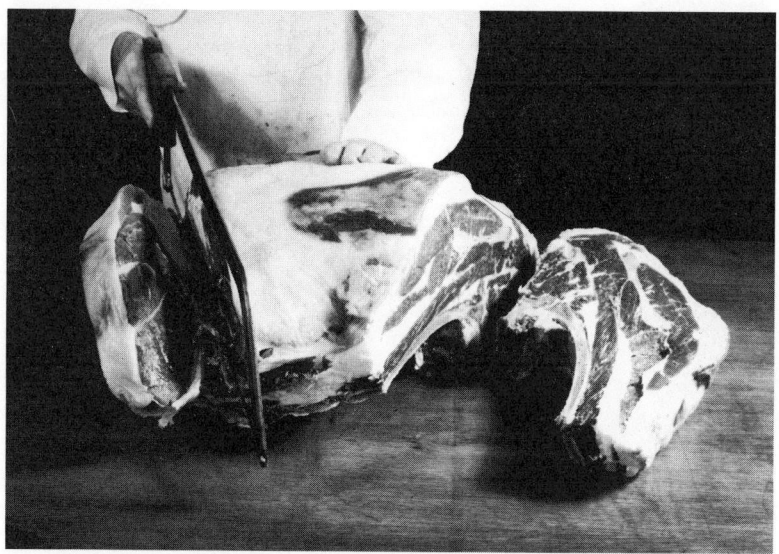

Fig. 36. Dividing chuck into steaks and pot roasts

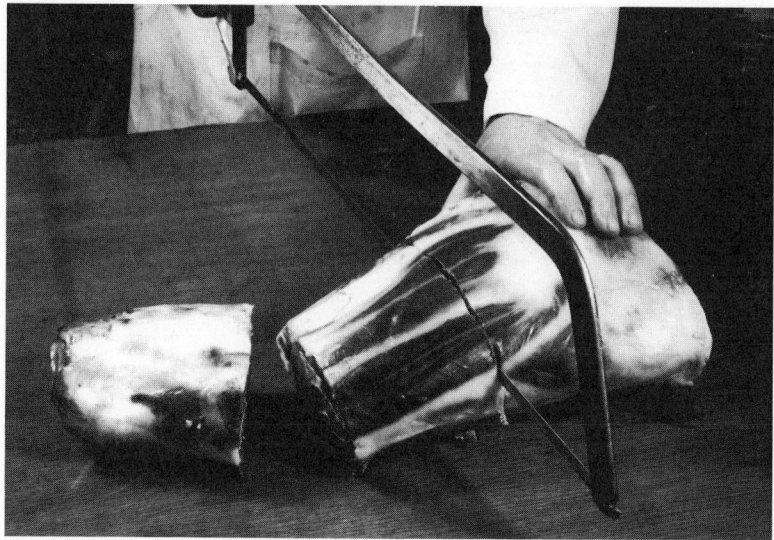

Fig. 37. Sawing foreshank into soup bones

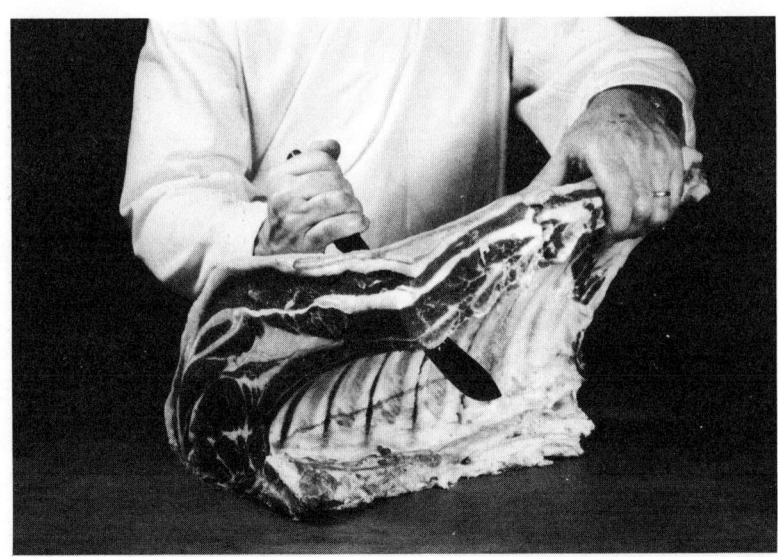

Fig. 38. Dividing prime rib into standing rib roasts

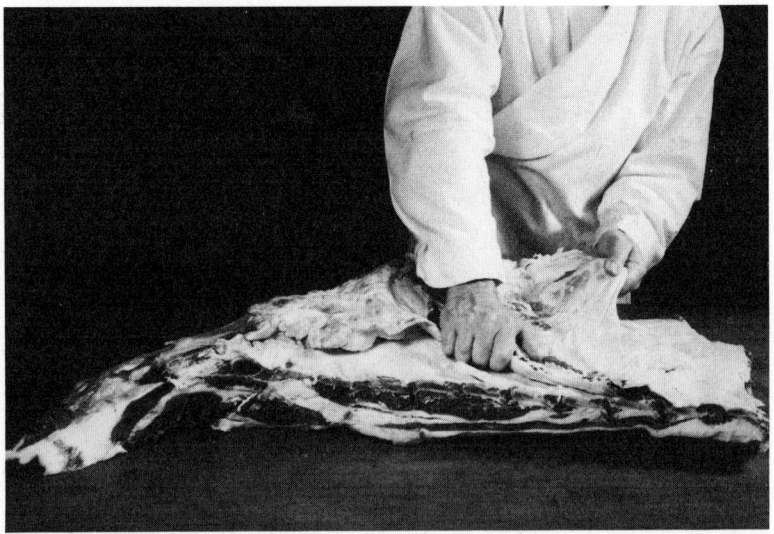

Fig. 39. Removing fascia from plate

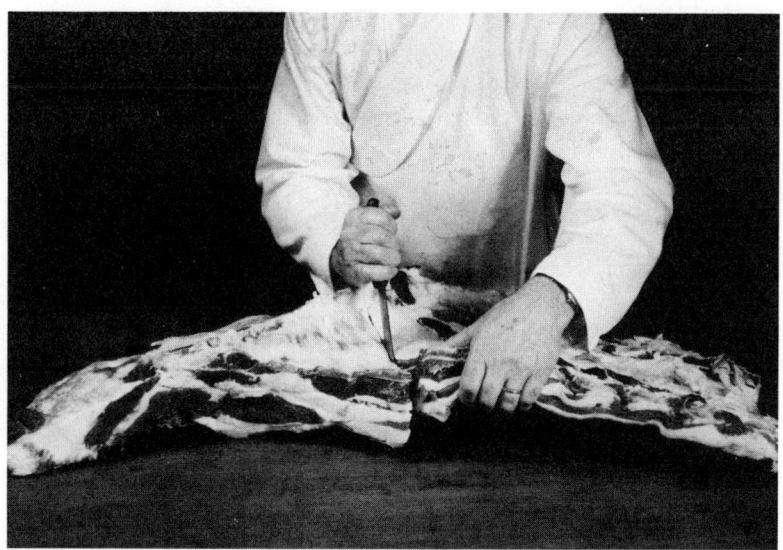

Fig. 40. Separating breast into plate and brisket

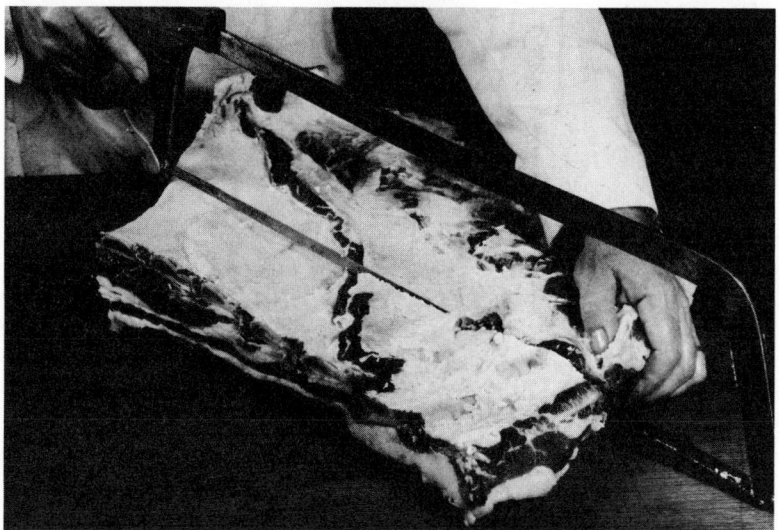

Fig. 41. Cutting plate into short ribs

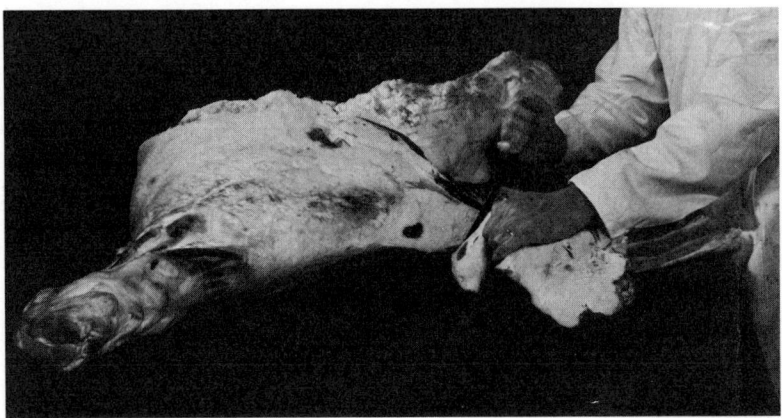

Fig. 42. Removing flank

YIELD

Approximate yields of trimmed quarters from an animal weighing 750 pounds and a dressed carcass weighing 420 pounds are as follows:

Trimmed quarters	Live weight (percent)	Carcass weight (percent)	Yield (pounds)
Hindquarters................	27.5	49.0	206
Forequarters	28.5	51.0	214
Total..................	56.0	100.00	420

Approximate yields of trimmed beef cuts from dressed forequarters weighing 214 pounds and dressed hindquarters weighing 206 pounds are as follows:

Trimmed cuts	Live weight (percent)	Carcass weight (percent)	Yield (pounds)
Steaks and oven roasts	23.0	41.0	172
Pot roasts..................	11.5	20.0	84
Stew and ground meat	11.5	20.0	84
Fat trim and bone	10.0	19.0	80
Total..................	56.0	100.00	420

THE HINDQUARTER

Lay the hindquarter on the table with the inside of the carcass up. Remove the flank by cutting from *10* to *1* (figs. 28 and 42). The cut at *10* should expose a small piece of lean. Remove the kidney knob by first cutting under the fat, then pulling the kidney knob out (fig. 43).

You are now ready to separate the loin from the round and rump. Do this by locating point *11,* which is about halfway between the tail head and the start of the rise of the pelvic arch, or about four sacral vertebrae. With a knife cut a straight line from this point (*11*) and about 1 inch in front of the aitch bone to the point at which the flank was removed (line *10* to *11,* fig. 28). After marking this line and cutting to the bone, saw through the bone and continue the separation with a knife. Use a knife to cut through the thick meaty portion, thus avoiding a rough irregular cut surface (fig. 44).

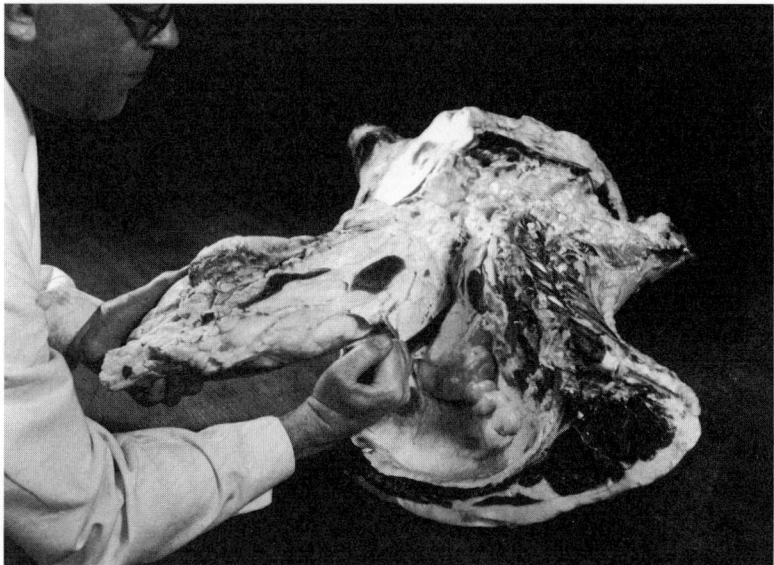

Fig. 43. Removing kidney knob and bed fat

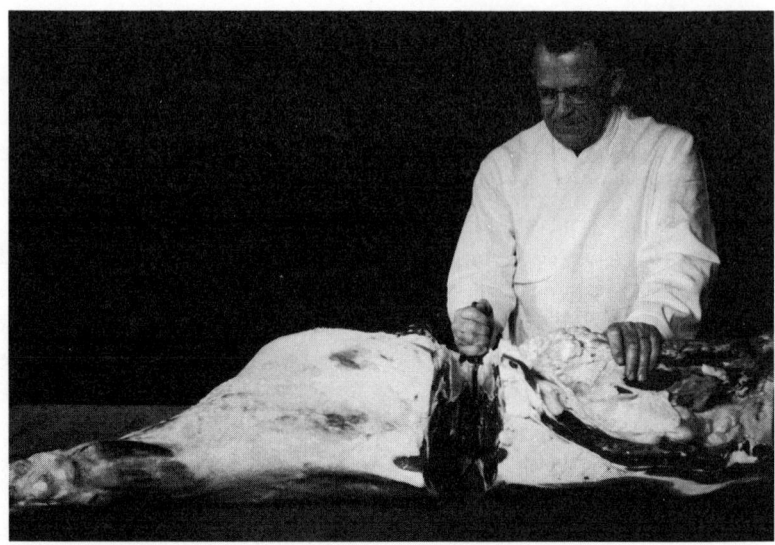

Fig. 44. Separating loin from round and rump

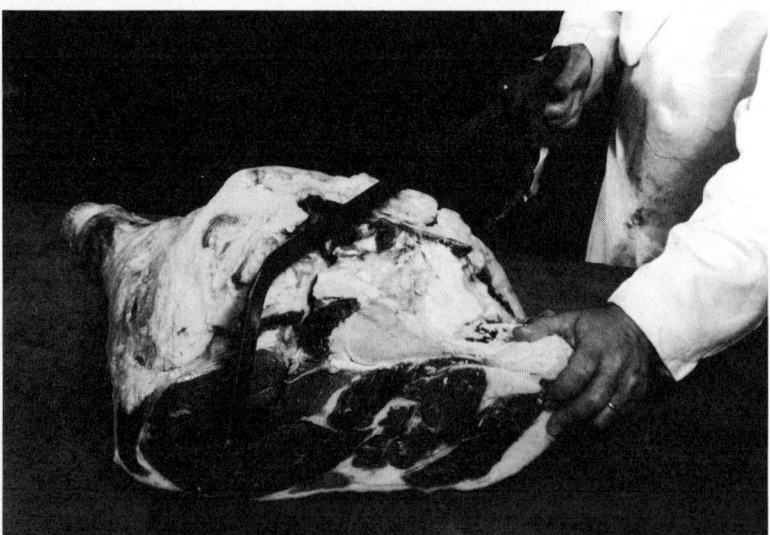

Fig. 45. Separating rump and round.

Separate the rump from the round by cutting on line *12* to *13* (fig. 28). Make this cut just back of and parallel to the pelvic bone, extending straight to either edge (fig. 45). Remove the hind shank by cutting through the meat to the bone on back of the shank, turning the knife up and following the bone to the joint (line *16* to *17,* fig. 28). Now, work the knife between the joint and finish the cut (fig. 46).

You are now ready to cut the hindquarters into usable pieces. Divide the loin, consisting of the short loin and loin end, along line *14* to *15* in figure 28 (figs. 47 and 48). The joint at which this separation starts is the cartilaginous end of the hip bone. These two cuts contain the club, porterhouse, and sirloin steaks. The porterhouse steaks are those that have a large portion of the tenderloin muscle (indicated by arrow in figure 49). Cut the steaks to the thickness you prefer.

Remove the kidney from the knob of fat by cutting through the fat to the kidney, being sure to cut the white membrane covering the kidney. With your hands, spread or break the fat apart and slip the kidney out (fig. 50).

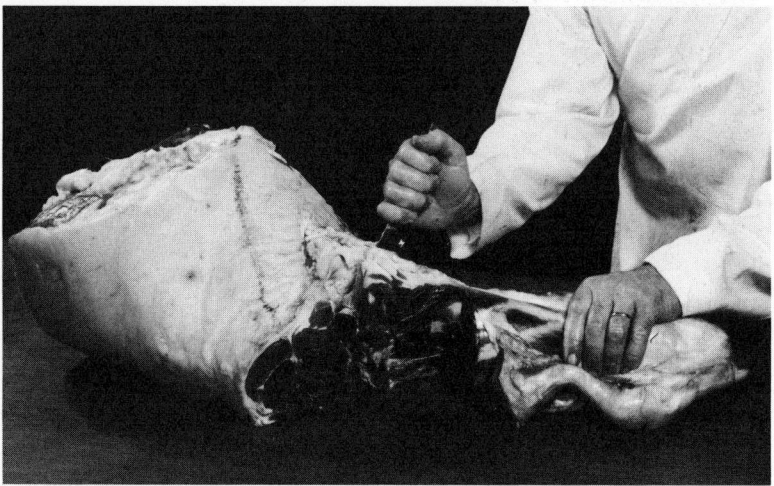

Fig. 46. Removing hind shank from round

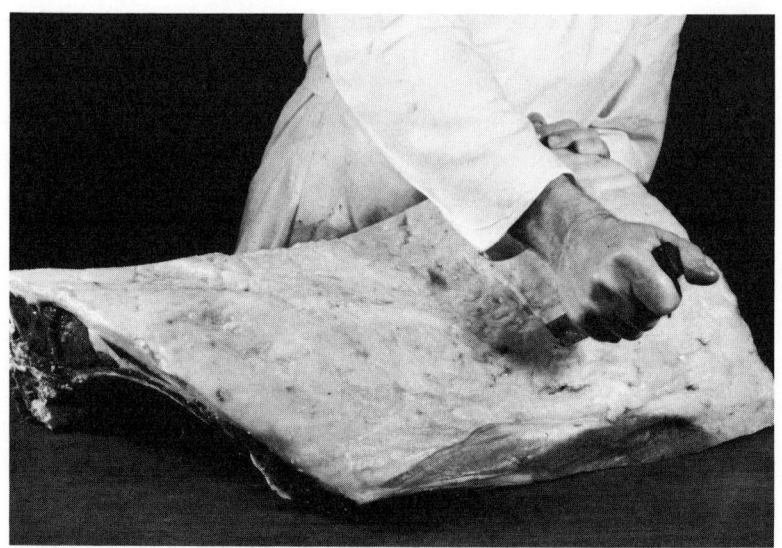

Fig. 47. Marking separation of short loin and loin end

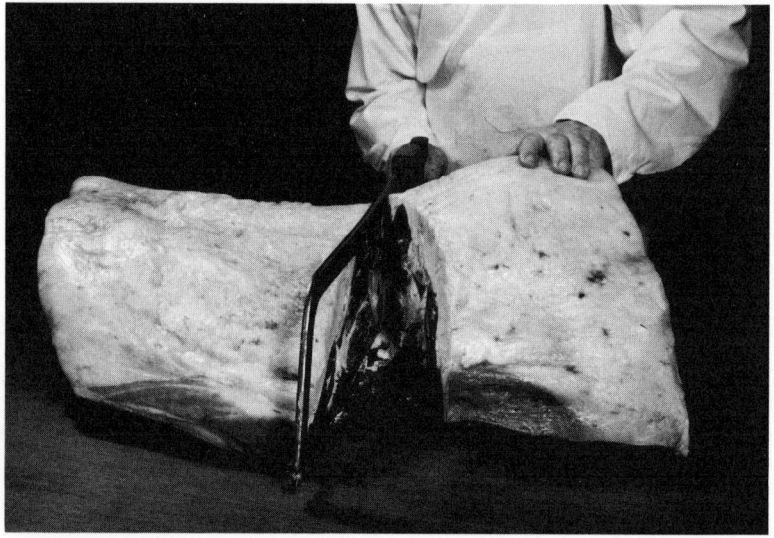

Fig. 48. Separating loin into short loin and loin end

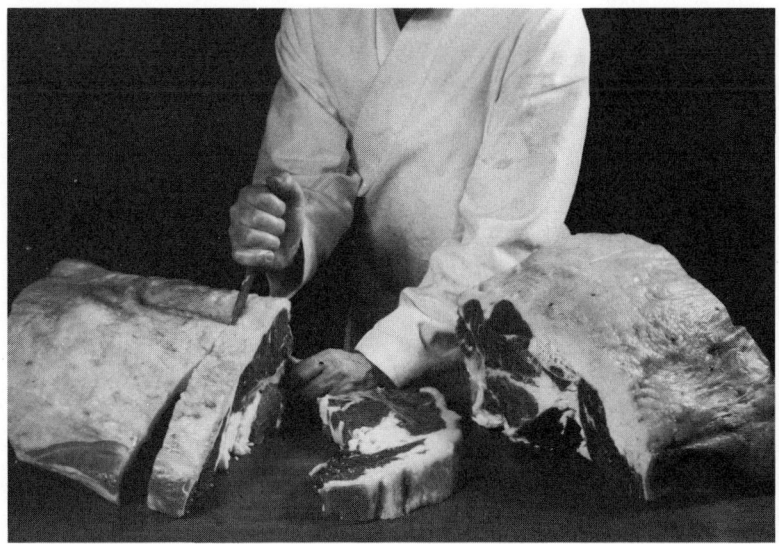

Fig. 49. Cutting porterhouse steaks from short loin

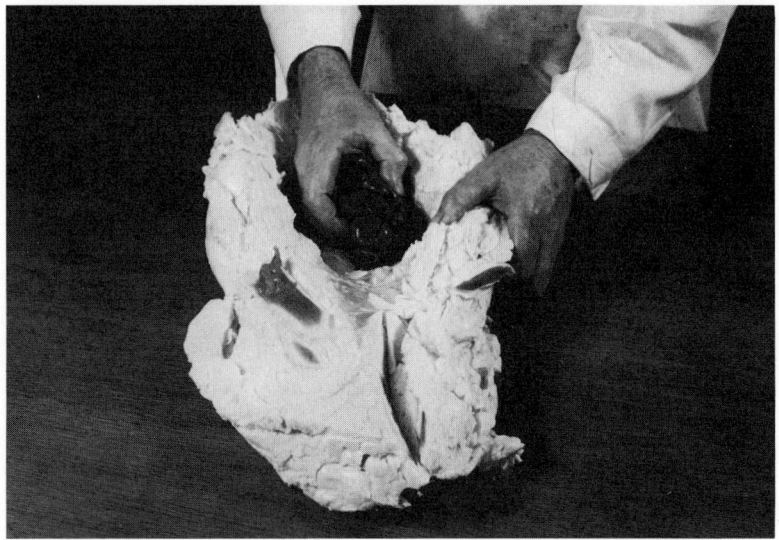

Fig. 50. Removing kidney from kidney knob or fat

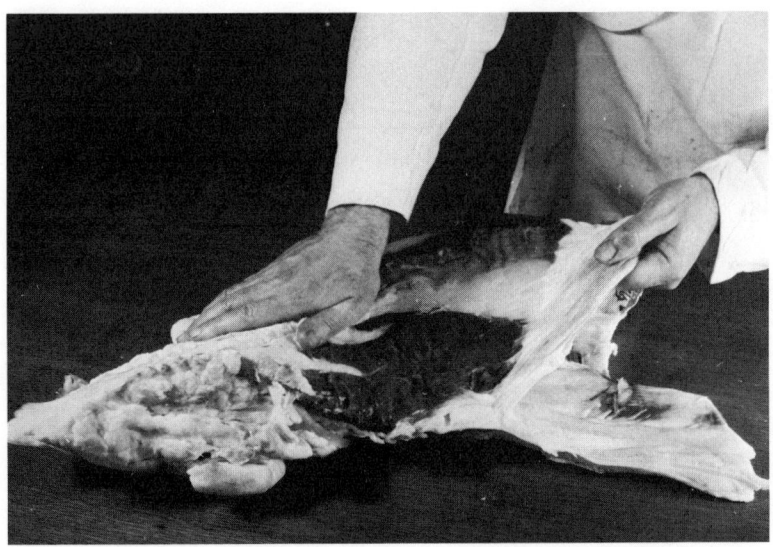

Fig. 51. Removing white membrane from lean of flank

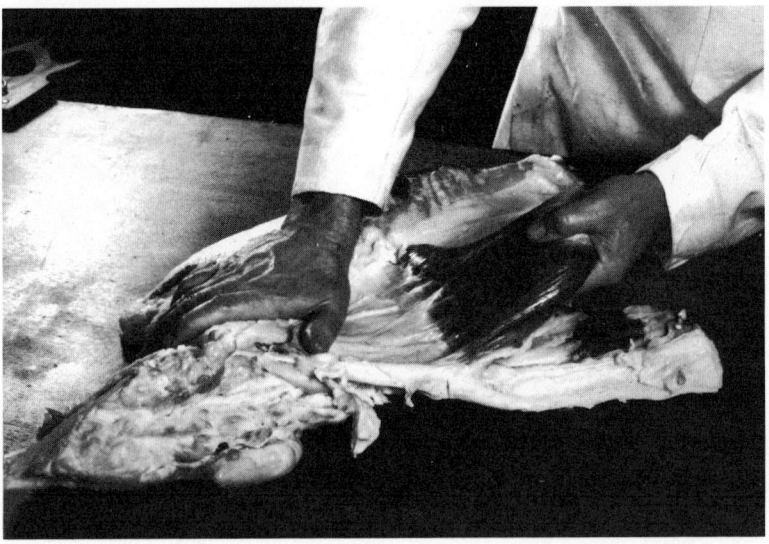

Fig. 51. Removing flank muscle from flank

You may separate the flank into fat and lean; grind the latter as hamburger, or remove the flank muscle and use it as flank steak. You must first pull the white tough covering from the lean muscle (fig. 51), then cut the small end loose and pull the muscle out (fig. 52). To use this muscle as a steak, lay it on the table and with a sharp knife divide it into two parts. Remove the aitch bone from the rump, then roll, tie, and trim the boneless rump. You can divide the round into three parts by following the seams between the large muscle. This gives the inside, outside, and a heel of round roast. If you prefer, you can cut steaks from the entire length of the round. However, you should cut the last 6 inches into small pieces for stew meat or grind for hamburger. You can handle the hindshank the same as the foreshank.

Processing

Fresh beef is perishable, and you should keep it under refrigeration temperatures from 34° to 36° F. at all times. Beef, unlike pork, can be improved by aging. However, it is advisable to allow the carcass to hang only about 7 days, then cut and process. If you desire additional aging, hold only the ribs, loins, and rounds for the additional time, which may vary from 1 to 6 or 7 weeks, the length of time depending on your preference. Aging does result in more tender meat and, if the beef is allowed to age long enough, a distinct flavor will develop. This characteristic flavor is desired by some and not by others. Only beef of the better grades should be considered for aging.

You can preserve farm beef in three ways: by freezing, curing, or canning. Each method results in a product that has its own characteristic flavor.

FREEZING[2]

Freezing beef does not improve its quality; therefore, use only beef of high quality. Tenderness is temporarily improved by freezing, although this is lost after 4 to 8 weeks of storage. To maintain the original quality, be sure to —

- Freeze only high-quality cuts.
- Prepare and freeze cuts promptly (not more than 15 days after slaughter).
- Prepare convenient, family-size packages.
- Protect meat from drying out (freezer burn) and oxidation by packaging in airtight and moisture-vapor resistant materials.
- Label and date each package.
- Freeze at — 10° F. or lower.
- Store at 0° F. or lower.
- Use ground meat within 4 months.
- Do not store frozen meat more than 12 months.

Frozen beef can be cooked thawed or unthawed. If you thaw meat before cooking, do it in a refrigerator. Cook thawed meat immediately or keep for only a short time in a refrigerator. Avoid refreezing thawed meat. If refreezing is necessary, do it promptly.

Any unthawed roast requires about one-third longer to cook than a thawed roast. Unthawed steaks may take about twice as long as thawed.

CURING

You can cure beef in two ways — by making it into corned

---

[2]For further information on freezing meat and fish in the home, consult your county agricultural agent or write to the U.S. Department of Agriculture, Washington, D.C. 20250.

beef or dried beef. Both methods use a combination of dry and brine curing in which salt, sugar, and saltpeter (potassium nitrate) are used.

CORNED BEEF

Corned beef is generally made from the cheaper cuts and those that have considerable fat, such as the plate, rump, and chuck.

Remove all bone from the cut and, to facilitate packing, cut pieces into uniform thickness and size. For each 100 pounds of meat, use 8 to 10 pounds of coarse salt. Spread a layer of salt on the bottom of a clean, sterilized wooden barrel or stone crock. Next, pack a layer of meat in the container; sprinkle with salt and add the next layer of meat and salt, and so on. Lightly rub each piece of meat with salt before packing. Allow the packed meat to stand for about 24 hours, at which time cover with a brine made up as follows: For each 100 pounds of meat, use 4 pounds of sugar, 4 ounces of saltpeter and 2 ounces of baking soda dissolved in 4 gallons of water. After covering with brine, weight the meat down.

High-quality corned beef requires from 30 to 40 days of curing. At the end of the curing period, remove the corned beef from the cure as needed, wash, and dry or smoke.

Keep a close watch on the brine as it may become ropy, especially if the temperatures rise much above 38° F. When this happens, remove the meat, wash thoroughly in warm water, repack in a new clean container (or in the original container, thoroughly washed and sterilized), and cover with new brine.

DRIED BEEF

Dried beef is made from the heavier-muscled cuts, especially the round. Cut the muscles lengthwise or prepare as a whole muscle. The curing procedure is the same as that used for corned beef except that you may add an extra pound of sugar for each 100 pounds of meat. After the meat is cured, remove it from the brine, wash, and hang up to dry for 24 hours. Smoke the cured meat in the regular manner at a temperature of 130° to 140° F. for 70 to 80 hours or until quite dry. The dried beef is ready to be used or it can be hung in a dry, dark room or wrapped and hung up for storage. Dried beef is usually cut very thin for use.

Smoking Beef. — Smoking cured meat probably aids in its preservation. It does give the meat a more desirable flavor and color, and dries it out more rapidly. The same smokehouse and procedures used for cured pork work well for beef.[3]

You may store smoked dried beef in the smokehouse if it is ventilated and free of flies. A cool, dry, dark and well-ventilated basement (free of flies) is a satisfactory storage area.

CANNING[4]

You can very satisfactorily preserve beef by canning if you do it properly. The most effective method is the steam-pressure canner, where sterilization temperature of 240° F. is obtained and can be held for the proper length of time. A water bath or a steamer without pressure does not result in a sufficiently high temperature to produce an effective sterilization.

Use only clean and sound beef for canning. You may can beef soon after chilling, as aging has little or no effect on the flavor or tenderness of canned meat. Remove all excess fat covering from beef before canning.

---

[3]For further information on slaughtering, cutting, and processing pork on the farm, consult your county agricultural agent or write to the U.S. Department of Agriculture, Washington, D.C. 20250.

[4]For detailed instructions on home canning of meats, consult your county agriculture agent or write to the U.S. Department of Agriculture, Washington, D.C. 22050.

Preparing Beef Products

PICKLING TRIPE

After you have thoroughly cleaned and rinsed the tripe in cold water, scald it in hot water (a little below the boiling point). When sufficiently scalded, remove the inside lining of the stomachs by scraping, which will leave a clean, white surface. Boil tripe until tender (usually about 3 hours) and then place in cold water so that you may scrape the fat from the outside. When you have done this, peel off the membrane from the outside of the stomach, and the clean, white tripe is ready for pickling.

Place the tripe in a clean, hardwood barrel or earthenware jar, and keep submerged in a strong brine for 3 or 4 days. Rinse with cold water and cover with pure cider vinegar or a spiced pickling liquid. Place a weight on the tripe to keep it from floating on the surface of the liquid.

MAKING HAMBURGER

Grind lean beef, such as the round, neck, flank, and trimmings, with a little fat, in a sausage grinder. If you desire, add a small amount of bacon for flavor. For seasoning, about 1 pound of salt and 4 ounces of pepper are sufficient for 50 pounds of meat.

MAKING BOLOGNA-STYLE SAUSAGE

In making bologna, for each 20 pounds of beef, add 5 pounds

of fresh pork. Grind the meat coarse, then add the seasoning and grind through the fine plate.

For seasoning 25 pounds of meat, ½ pound of salt, and 2½ ounces of pepper are usually satisfactory. Garlic may be added if desired.

Add 3 to 4 pints of water to this quantity of meat. Mix with the hands until the water is entirely absorbed by the meat. When thoroughly mixed, stuff into soaked beef casings or "rounds," and smoke the bologna from 2 to 3 hours at a temperature of from 60° to 70°F.

After smoking, cook the bologna in water about 200° F., or slightly below the boiling point, until it floats.

Keep the sausage in a dry place for immediate use, or can it by packing in cans, covering to within one-half inch of top with the liquid in which the bologna was cooked. Then heat it to a temperature of 250° F. for 45 minutes, or at 15 pounds steam pressure.

SHIPPING FARM MEAT INTERSTATE

Farmers who ship their meats must comply with State and Federal regulations. For details about these regulations, consult your county agricultural agent or write to the U.S. Department of Agriculture, Washington, D.C. 20250.

Handling The Hide

Remove dirt, blood, and any pieces of flesh on the hide by scraping with the back of a butcher knife and by careful cutting. Allow the hide to lose its animal heat before applying salt. When the hide was cooled sufficiently, spread it, hair side down, being sure to straighten out all folds and laps. Sprinkle fresh, clean salt over the flesh side of the hide, using about 1 pound for every pound of hide. See that all parts of the flesh side receive a sprinkling of the salt. Be sure to use plenty of salt and rub it in well along cut edges, head, neck, legs, wrinkles, and the heavy portions.[5]

Slaughtering Calves

Most veal is produced in this country from calves between 1 and 3 months old, weighing from 160 to 200 pounds.

Stun the calf before sticking it (as in killing cattle), but the blow need not be heavy. The work is made easier if you hoist the carcass to a convenient height before skinning. Wash the hide and split the skin from head to tail, following the middle line of the belly. If you cut the carcass on the farm, remove the hide at once, as the carcass can be skinned more easily while it is still warm. Use a knife to start the skin, then "fist" off the hide. Remove the offal, and split the breastbone and pelvis, as described for beef.

Most veal calves have little or no outside fat covering. Cut and process the carcass and meat as soon as possible to avoid dark, dried surfaces and excessive loss of moisture.

Cut and process veal carcasses the same as with the beef carcass. Because of the lack of finish, do not make corned beef or drief beef from veal or calf meat.

---

[5]For detailed instructions on proper handling of beef hides, consult your county agricultural agent or write to the U.S. Department of Agriculture, Washington, D.C. 20250.

This bulletin supersedes Farmers' Bulletin 1415, "Beef on the Farm—Slaughtering, Cutting, Curing."

Appendix

GROWTH TABLE FOR WEIGHT AND HEIGHT OF FEMALE DAIRY CALVES

Age (months)	Holstein Weight (pounds)	Holstein Withers height (inches)	Ayrshire Weight (pounds)	Ayrshire Withers height (inches)	Jersey Weight (pounds)	Jersey Withers height (inches)
Birth	90	29.0	72	27.6	55	25.7
1	115	30.5	89	28.6	70	27.0
2	155	32.2	119	30.2	95	28.8
3	205	34.3	158	31.9	135	30.6
4	260	36.3	198	34.0	175	32.7
5	318	37.7	245	35.5	220	34.5
6	380	39.5	293	37.2	270	36.1
7	438	41.2	344	38.5	315	37.6
8	490	42.5	389	39.9	360	39.0
9	543	43.6	433	40.9	395	40.0
10	590	44.5	469	41.7	430	41.0
11	635	45.2	502	42.5	465	41.8
12	685	46.0	538	43.2	495	42.4
14	753	47.5	611	44.8	550	43.5
16	820	48.6	669	45.7	600	44.6
18	890	49.5	725	46.5	645	45.4
20	960	50.5	793	47.4	695	46.2

Adapted from Missouri Agricultural Experimental Station data, Bulletin 336, 1934, by A. C. Ragsdale, and data from other sources.

ESTIMATION OF COW'S WEIGHT ACCORDING TO HEART GIRTH

Circ. of Chest (in.)	Wt. in lbs.	Circ. of Chest (in.)	Wt. in lbs.	Circ. of Chest (in.)	Wt. in lbs.
30.0	100	51.0	414	72.0	1064
30.5	103	51.5	424	72.5	1085
31.0	107	52.0	434	73.0	1104
31.5	112	52.5	445	73.5	1126
32.0	117	53.0	456	74.0	1146
32.5	121	53.5	467	74.5	1169
33.0	127	54.0	476	75.0	1191
33.5	131	54.5	495	75.5	1213
34.0	137	55.0	510	76.0	1236
34.5	141	55.5	521	76.5	1263
35.0	146	56.0	534	77.0	1285
35.5	152	56.5	545	77.5	1308
36.0	157	57.0	562	78.0	1331
36.5	162	57.5	577	78.5	1354
37.0	167	58.0	590	79.0	1377
37.5	173	58.5	605	79.5	1400
38.0	179	59.0	616	80.0	1423
38.5	186	59.5	629	80.5	1446
39.0	193	60.0	647	81.0	1469
39.5	199	60.5	668	81.5	1492
40.0	206	61.0	684	82.0	1515
40.5	214	61.5	700	82.5	1538
41.0	223	62.0	716	83.0	1561
41.5	229	62.5	732	83.5	1584
42.0	239	63.0	748	84.0	1607
42.5	247	63.5	762	84.5	1629
43.0	255	64.0	778	85.0	1650
43.5	270	64.5	790	85.5	1673
44.0	283	65.0	815	86.0	1692
44.5	293	65.5	828	86.5	1718
45.0	298	66.0	848	87.0	1741
45.5	307	66.5	866	87.5	1764
46.0	315	67.0	883	88.0	1788
46.5	323	67.5	891	88.5	1812
47.0	334	68.0	904	89.0	1833
47.5	344	68.5	923	89.5	1857
48.0	354	69.0	942	90.0	1881
48.5	364	69.5	962	90.5	1905
49.0	374	70.0	982	91.0	1929
49.5	384	70.5	1002	91.5	1952
50.0	394	71.0	1022	92.0	1975
50.5	404	71.5	1043		

FEED ANALYSIS TABLE (As-Fed Basis*)

	Dry Matter %	Crude Protein %	TDN %	Fiber %	Ca %	P %
DRY ROUGHAGES						
Alfalfa	90	15.5	51	29	1.5	0.2
Bromegrass (bloom)	90	8.5	49	28	0.4	0.2
Mixed hay, good,						
M30% legumes	90	9.0	49	31	1.0	0.2
Oat Straw	90	4.0	45	36	0.24	0.1
Ochard grass	90	8.0	49	30	0.25	0.2
Prairie hay						
(midseason)	90	6.0	45	—	0.3	0.1
Quack grass	90	7.0	40	35	—	—
Timothy, good	90	6.5	49	30	0.35	0.14
Timothy, late	90	5.5	41	31	0.14	0.15
Timothy & ¼						
clover	90	8.0	50	30	0.58	0.15
Corn fodder	80	7.0	55	21	0.25	0.14
Corn stover	80	6.0	45	27	0.48	0.08
SUCCULENTS						
Apples, whole	18	0.5	13	1.5	0.01	0.01
Apple pomace	21	1.5	16	4.0	0.02	0.02
Cabbage	9.5	2.0	8	1.0	0.06	0.03
Carrots	12	1.0	10.5	1.0	0.05	0.04
Corn silage	27	2.5	18.5	7.0	0.1	0.07
Kale	12	2.5	8	1.5	0.2	0.06
Mangels	10	1.5	7	1.0	0.02	0.02
Potatoes	21	2.0	17.5	0.5	0.01	0.05
Rutabaga, (Swede)	11	1.5	9.5	1.5	0.05	0.03
Sorghum silage	25.5	1.5	15	7.0	0.08	0.05
Sweet potatoes	31	1.5	25.5	2.0	0.03	0.04
Pumpkins	10	2.0	9	2.0	—	—
Sugar Beet (tops)	16	1.5	14	1.0	0.03	0.07
Turnips	10	1.0	8	2.0	0.06	0.02
GRAINS						
Barley	89	13	77	5.5	0.06	0.35
Corn	88	9	83	2.0	0.02	0.30
Oats (whole)	90	12	70	12.0	0.09	0.30
Sorghum	89	11	80	2.0	0.05	0.30
PASTURE						
Mixed grasses	20	4	15	6.0	0.60	0.30

FEED ANALYSIS TABLE (As-Fed Basis*) (Continued)

	Dry Matter %	Crude Protein %	TDN %	Fiber %	Ca %	P %
PROTEIN SUPPLEMENTS						
Cottonseed meal	91	41	70	11	0.15	1.1
Corn gluten meal	91	43	80	4	0.16	0.40
Linseed oil meal	91	35	73	9	0.40	0.80
Wheat bran	89	16	66	10	0.10	1.2
Wheat middlings	90	18	78	4	0.10	0.80
COMMERCIAL CONCENTRATE						
premixed	90	12-22	70-75	11	0.60	0.50

* Meaning that in order to calculate nutrient values of these feeds you simply multiply the percentage CP or TDN times the total weight of food being fed or being consumed. In other tables you may find CP and TDN values given under the heading *Dry Matter Basis*. In that case it is necessary first to find out the dry matter content of the weight of the feed being fed or consumed before going on to calculate your CP, TDN or other values. From *The Family Cow*, Garden Way Publishing.

SEEDING RATES AND ESTIMATED ACRE YIELDS

Seed	Bushel Weight		Seed per Acre	Yield per Acre
Corn	50-56	drilled	1¼-2¼ bu.	20 tons (green)
Cabbage	50-56	drill or transplant	4-6 lbs.	20 tons
Carrot	30	drilled	6-8 lbs.	15 tons
Kale	50	drill or broadcast	2-6 lbs. 10 lbs.	20 tons
Kohlrabi	50-56	drilled	3-5 lbs.	15 tons
Mangel	50	drilled	5-7 lbs.	30-40 tons
Parsnip	17-19	drilled	6-8 lbs.	12-15 tons
Potato	56	hills	1500 lbs.	10-15 tons
Rape	50	drilled broadcast	2-6 lbs.	12-15 tons
Sugar Beet	16-20	drilled	12 lbs.	12-20 tons
Swede (Rutabaga)	50-56	drilled	3-4 lbs.	15-20 tons
Sweet Potato		slips or cuttings	6 bu.	90-200 bu.

ESTIMATING GRAINS AND ROUGHAGES

1. **To find the number of bushels of grain or shelled corn in a bin:** Obtain total cubic feet of grain by multiplying the length by the width by the average depth (all in feet). Divide by 1¼ (or multiply by 0.8) to find bushels. Round bin—multiply distance around the bin by the diameter by the depth of grain (all in feet) and divide by 5.

2. **To find the number of bushels of ear corn in crib:** Rectangular crib—multiply the length by the width by the average depth (all in feet) and divide by 2½ (or multiply by 0.4) to find bushels. Round crib—multiply the distance around the crib by the diameter by the depth of the corn (all in feet) and divide by 10.

3. **To find tons of loose hay in mow:** Multiply the length by the width by the height (all in feet) and divide by 400 to 525, depending on the kind of hay and how long it has been in the mow.

4. **To find tons of loose hay in stack:** Rectangular stacks—secure the overthrow, O (the distance from the ground, close to stack, on one side over the top of the stack to the ground on the other side); the width, W; and the length, L (all in feet). Additional rules for round stacks will be found on page 4 of U.S.D.A. Leaflet No. 72, published in February, 1931.

   The contents in cubic feet may then be determined as follows:

   (a) For low round-topped stacks
   $$[(.52 \times O) - (.44 \times W)] \times W \times L$$
   (b) For high round-topped stacks
   $$[(.52 \times O) - (.46 \times W)] \times W \times L$$

Divide the number of cubic feet thus secured by the follow cubic feet allowed per ton:

When settled:	1 to 3 months	Over 3 months
Alfalfa Hay	485	470
Timothy	640	625
Wild Hay	600	450

For clover hay use about the same as alfalfa or slightly higher (500 to 512).

5. **To find the number of tons of straw:** Follow the same method as is used with hay except that about twice as many cubic feet (900 to 1,000) are allowed per ton.

6. **Fodder and stover** are usually estimated on the acre basis, estimating the amount of corn in the fodder and allowing some additional value per acre for the stover.

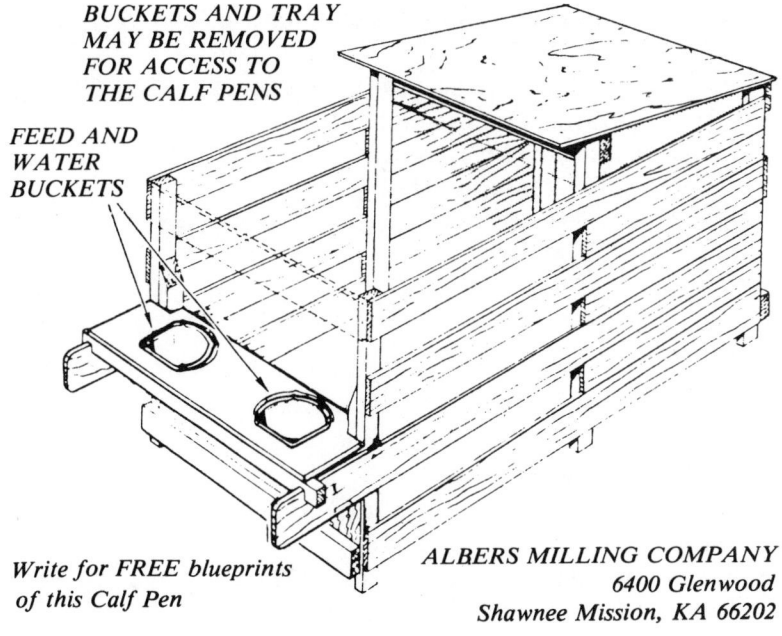

BUCKETS AND TRAY
MAY BE REMOVED
FOR ACCESS TO
THE CALF PENS

FEED AND
WATER
BUCKETS

*Write for FREE blueprints
of this Calf Pen*

ALBERS MILLING COMPANY
6400 Glenwood
Shawnee Mission, KA 66202

CATTLE ASSOCIATIONS
Registered Dairy Cattle:
The American Dairy Cattle Club. Robert W. Hitchcock, Interlaken, NY 14847.

The American Guernsey Cattle Club. 70 Main Street, Peterborough, NH 03458.

The American Jersey Cattle Club. 2105 J South Hamilton Rd., Columbus, OH 43227.

The American Red Danish Cattle Association. Marlette, MI 48453.

The Ayrshire Breeders' Association. Box 1038, Beloit, WI 53511.

The Holstein-Friesian Association of America. Box 808, Brattleboro, VT 05301.

Red and White Dairy Cattle Association. Box 771, Elgin, IL 60120.

The Canadian Cattle Breeders' Society (Societe des Eleveurs de Bovins Canadiens). Roxton Pond (Shefford), Quebec JOE 1ZO, Canada.

The Purebred Dairy Cattle Association. 70 Main St., Peterborough, NH 03458.

Ayrshire Breeders' Association of Canada, 1160 Carling Ave., Ottawa, Ontario, K1Z 7K6.

Canadian Brown Swiss Association, 358 Wellington St., St. Thomas, Ontario, N5R 2T5.

Canadian Jersey Cattle Club, 343 Waterloo Ave., Guelph, Ontario, N1M 3K1.

Canadian Guernsey Breeders' Association, 368 Woolrich St., Guelph, Ontario.

Holstein-Friesian Association of Canada, Brantford, Ontario.

Dual-Purpose Cattle:
The American Milking Shorthorn Society. 313 South Glenstone Ave., Springfield, MO.

Red Poll Cattle Club of America. 3275 Holdrege St., Lincoln, NE.

Canadian Shorthorn Association, 5 Douglas Street, Guelph, Ontario, N1H 2S8.
Canadian Red Poll Cattle Association, Francis, Saskatchewan, SOG 1VO.

METRIC EQUIVALENTS

Length

inch	= 2.54 cm	millimetre	= 0.039 in
foot	= 0.3048 m	centimetre	= 0.394 in
yard	= 0.914 m	decimetre	= 3.937 in
mile	= 1.609 km	metre	= 3.28 ft
		kilometre	= 0.621 mile

Area

square inch	= 6.452 cm^2	cm^2	= 0.155 sq in
square foot	= 0.093 m^2	m^2	= 1.196 sq yd
square yard	= 0.836 m^2	km^2	= 0.386 sq mile
square mile	= 2.59 km^2	ha	= 2.471 ac
acre	= 0.405 ha		

Volume (Dry)

cubic inch	= 16.387 cm^3	cm^3	= 0.061 cu in
cubic foot	= 0.028 m^3	m^3	= 31.338 cu ft
cubic yard	= 0.765 m^3	hectolitre	= 2.8 bu
bushel	= 36.368 litres	m^3	= 1.308 cu yd
board foot	= 0.0024 m^3		

Volume (Liquid)

fluid ounce (Imp)	= 28.412 ml	litre	= 35.2 fluid oz
pint	= 0.568 litre	hectolitre	= 26.418 gal
gallon	= 4.546 litres		

Weight

ounce	= 28,349 g	gram	= 0.035 oz avdp
pound	= 453.592 g	kilogram	= 2.205 lb avdp
hundredweight (Imp)	= 45.359 kg	tonne	= 1.102 short ton
ton	= 0.907 tonne		

Proportion

1 gal/acre	= 11.232 litres/ha	1 litre/ha	= 14.24 fluid oz/acre
1 lb/acre	= 1.120 kg/ha	1 kg/ha	= 14.5 oz avdp/acre
1 lb/sq in	= 0.0702 kg/cm^2	1 kg/cm^2	= 14.227 lb/sq in
1 bu/acre	= 00.098 hl/ha	1 hl/ha	= 1.112 bu/acre

Index